Contents

About the authors

Alan Chapman worked as a social work practitioner and in staff development prior to becoming Education and Training Officer at the Dementia Centre in 1991. He has co-written and edited a number of training publications, and provides in-house dementia education programmes for care home and day care staff.

Donna Gilmour trained as a nurse but moved to be deputy manager of a specialist 30-place social services department dementia care home for five years. In April 2000, she became manager of a voluntary organisation care home in Edinburgh.

Iain McIntosh is a retired family doctor and hospital practitioner, who specialised in the rehabilitation of older people and people with dementia. He is currently a lecturer at Stirling and Glasgow Universities. He is an audit and GP training assessor with the Scottish Council for Post Graduate Medical Education, and has written a book on dementia management for GPs.

Dementia Care

A professional handbook

Alan Chapman, Donna Gilmour
and Iain McIntosh

second edition

© 2001 Alan Chapman
Published by Age Concern England
1268 London Road
London SW16 4ER

First published 1994
Second edition published 2001

Editor   Sue Henning
Production   Vinnette Marshall
Design and typesetting   GreenGate Publishing Services
Printed in Great Britain by Bell & Bain Ltd, Glasgow

A catalogue record for this book is available from the British Library

ISBN 0-86242-313-9

Whilst the advice and information contained in *Dementia Care* is believed to be true and accurate at the time of going to press, neither Age Concern England nor the authors can accept any legal responsibility or liability for any errors or omissions that may be made.

Bulk orders
Age Concern England is pleased to offer customised editions of all its titles to UK companies, institutions or other organisations wishing to make a bulk purchase. For further information, please contact the Publishing Department at the address on this page. Tel: 020 8765 7200. Fax: 020 8765 7211. Email: books@ace.org.uk

Acknowledgements

The authors express their thanks to:

Mary Marshall, Director, Dementia Services Development Centre, University of Stirling, for the material used in Chapter 5.

Sally Knocker, Dementia – Staff Development and Resource Worker, Royal Borough of Kensington and Chelsea Social Services, London, for the case study material used in Chapter 6, and for her assistance in reviewing the final manuscript.

Bill McLean, Consultant Geriatrician, Taree, NSW, Australia, for the material used in Chapter 8.

Age Concern staff in the Legal and the Information and Policy departments for their help in reviewing the manuscript.

Introduction

A changing scene

The world of dementia care has seen many changes in the last five years. The traditional view that nothing can be done for the person has changed with the emergence of new drug treatments for Alzheimer's disease. Early detection and diagnosis are now of crucial importance. Equally significant is the greater understanding of the experience of dementia for individuals and the recognition that meaningful participation in everyday activity is possible.

There is also now a greater awareness of the impact of dementia on families and partners, and their need for information and education about dementia, as well as being involved in discussions concerning ongoing plans of action. Cultural differences are being recognised in the development of new services and support. General Practitioners (GPs) play a crucial role, as they are the first point of contact for most families, they can access specialist medical services and refer patients for community support or assessment for care homes.

As people with dementia are enabled to live at home longer, those coming in to care homes or day care may have more diverse and complex needs. The same is true for residents already living in care homes, who, over time, have developed dementia. Consequently, staff increasingly have to meet the differing and changing needs of residents with dementia and cope with often highly stressful situations, which require understanding, tolerance and insight. Where the home has a policy of not transferring residents with dementia to specialist hospital wards or dementia units, staff will be required to develop skills in sensitively supporting residents in the advanced stages of the illness.

Against the backdrop of these changes, there is also a greater emphasis on day care and respite care. As well as meeting in church halls, community centres or residential homes, day care groups can also meet in a carer's own home or that of a person with dementia. Respite care may mean an outreach worker from the local care home going to stay in the person's own home or the family member being enabled to drop the person off for a two-hour break at the home or day centre. Whatever the circumstances, working with people with dementia presents staff with three challenges:

CHALLENGE 1: SEE THE PERSON BEHIND THE LABEL OF DEMENTIA

The medical view that dementia is an impairment of brain function – which, over time, may rob the person of their ability to cope – is only part of the picture. The personal history, life experiences, relationships, cultural identity, personality and environment of each individual exert a potentially stronger influence than any dementia. Seeing the person first means that responses to the person with dementia require a heightened awareness, a sensitive approach and an insight concerning their life experiences. No two people with dementia are the same.

CHALLENGE 2: PROVIDE SUPPORT THAT MAINTAINS ABILITIES

The support given to people with dementia should encourage them to continue their ordinary, daily routines and activities, so that they are not restricted or forced prematurely into dependency. Underpinning all work with people with dementia should be the core values of:

- **maximising personal control:** believing the person has the right to opportunities to use whatever abilities they retain;
- **enabling choice:** actively encouraging communication and expression of individuality;
- **respecting dignity:** recognising that self-worth and self-esteem are part of overall health and wellbeing;
- **preserving continuity:** remembering that the person has a past, present and future;
- **promoting equity:** creating opportunities that are non-ageist and non-discriminatory.

CHALLENGE 3: OFFER CONTINUITY AND CREATIVE RESPONSES

Continuity of support means that attention is given to having a consistent and coherent response to the individual. Shift changes or the variability of volunteers should not lead to differences in what is seen as important. A familiar face can be crucial in alleviating anxiety for the person with dementia. Staff who recognise the importance of a caring relationship will adopt positive, creative responses, which actively involve residents and promote their individuality.

Essentially, dementia care is about understanding and being understood. This is a shared problem for those with dementia and for those who work with them. The person with dementia needs to be understood in terms of an illness that can create anxiety, uncertainty, insecurity and an acute sensitivity to their environment. Care staff face the challenge of helping the person make sense of what they experience and what is being said to them.

This second edition is firmly based on the belief that our past life experiences are significantly important. The memories and feelings associated with these experiences stay with us. They influence our behaviour, the routines we adopt, our attitude to others and how we cope with the here and now. It is at this level that we share a common bond with the person with dementia.

A basic assumption of this book is that the quality of life for people with dementia and their carers should be maintained at the highest possible level. The King's Fund has drawn up the following list of principles that are important in providing care and should be considered by all staff.

PEOPLE WITH DEMENTIA HAVE THE SAME HUMAN VALUE AS ANYONE ELSE, IRRESPECTIVE OF THEIR DEGREE OF DISABILITY OR INDEPENDENCE

Each of us, as members of society, have quite definite ideas about what is 'right' and 'wrong' and what we consider is 'acceptable' and 'unacceptable' about the behaviour of others. People who do not work, who are from another culture or who have a serious disability, risk being undervalued by us. Women, too, are often undervalued. Those who do not fit our idea of what is 'normal' or 'acceptable' can be subject to low expectations, discrimination and blame for the situation they are in. Many people with dementia experience these three judgements.

Our expectations about quality of life for people with dementia ought not to fall below the standards of other members of the community. Being 84 years of age and with a diagnosis of Alzheimer's, for example, should not lead staff to treat that person as an object of care. Each individual with dementia is unique and someone who can be enabled to maintain their ability and independence.

PEOPLE WITH DEMENTIA HAVE THE SAME VARIED NEEDS AS ANYONE ELSE

This means not only basic needs for food, warmth, shelter and protection from physical hurt but also affection, companionship, and opportunities to take part in meaningful activities. Re-read Challenge 2 on page vii. Only when people with dementia have access to the same range of human contact and resources that we experience can we hope to achieve support that recognises individuality, and social and emotional wellbeing. To help those with more severe dementia to enjoy the benefits of community life requires a high level of long-term support, professional skill, imagination and resources.

PEOPLE WITH DEMENTIA HAVE THE SAME RIGHTS AS OTHER CITIZENS

People with dementia are often denied opportunities and access to resources to which they have a right. In many situations, it is because the person is seen as being unable to assert their just demands or express choice.

Given the opportunity, most people with dementia can express their feelings and are well able to communicate displeasure, pain or their opinion. Care workers should seek ways to make claims on their behalf and strive to preserve their rights. In following steps to change the legal status of an individual, the safeguards and access to representation should equate with the highest standards expected by other citizens.

EVERY PERSON IS AN INDIVIDUAL

Like anyone else, people with dementia have the right to express their own preferences, abilities and needs within the law. Look again at Challenge 2 on page vii and Challenge 3 on page viii. Individuality means having continuity between your past, your present and your future.

PEOPLE WITH DEMENTIA HAVE THE RIGHT TO FORMS OF SUPPORT THAT DO NOT EXPLOIT FAMILY AND FRIENDS

In many instances, partners, relatives, friends and neighbours provide the major source of support for people with dementia. Caring for someone 24 hours a day, 7 days a week, is stressful and exhausting. Care workers should ensure that they actively recognise the important role carried out by these carers and seek to give practical advice and support.

Many family carers experience feelings of guilt, loss and helplessness as they see the person with dementia change. The needs and wishes of the person with dementia may conflict with their carers, so staff should ensure that the rights of both are safeguarded.

Using the book

This book is aimed at care home managers and day centre organisers, and their staff (both paid and voluntary). It discusses important aspects associated with providing support to people with dementia. It also draws on the results of recent research and the authors' work experiences with people with dementia and those working with them. All of the incidents recorded actually happened but not necessarily in one care home or day care group.

The second edition has been written to update the original content, and also to stress a more holistic approach to the support of people with dementia: in essence, dementia, as an illness, does not rob the person of the influence of their past life. There are suggested training exercises linked to case studies, which are contained at the end of each chapter. These are intended to help readers develop their own ideas and thoughts on the issues raised. Suggested responses are included in Appendix 2.

Time management

This book does not have to be read at one sitting. Instead, it is recommended that you take time to go through it, spending about 20–30 minutes on each chapter, perhaps making brief notes as you go. Staff meetings can be used to discuss the questions posed in the exercises at the end of each chapter. A proposed timetable for short training sessions can be found in Appendix 1.

1 The individual and their previous lifestyle

Objectives:

- *To encourage readers to see the person first before the illness*
- *To highlight the impact on the individual of group care*

'When I look there (pointing at the window) the postcard is strange, it's not how it should be – where am I? If things were just in order.'

Miss Greene, who spoke these words, had just moved, two days previously, from the cottage where she had lived for 25 years to the new purpose-built nursing home for people with dementia. Her words tell us something about how she was feeling about the move into unfamiliar surroundings. Outwardly she seemed settled – she did not show any agitated behaviour – yet she was troubled. The view from the window was not the one that she had been familiar with over the past 25 years.

Life for people with dementia, like Miss Greene, did not begin on the day that they walked into the care home or day centre. Her unique life experiences, relationships, work experiences, the local community of which she was part and her immediate environment all combined to influence her. She had a routine that was familiar to her and created a feeling of security; suddenly she was in a strange, new place with faces that she did not recognise. Miss Greene then had to rely on this new environment and the people in it to provide her with a sense of security – to help her feel physically safe and not threatened, and to maintain a sense of self-worth and individuality.

It is crucial to recognise that the person with dementia, despite the effects of the illness, still has similar responses to coping with change, as do those without dementia. Staff members who understand this can gain an insight into reasons for the particular behaviour of individuals with dementia.

As individuals, our sense of self is the coming together of our personality, past experiences, routines and habits, relationships with others and feeling of being capable. Each one of us is different and our life experiences vary. The person with dementia is no different. The diversity of their life experiences means that each person is influenced by the illness in different ways. Their response to group care will also be different.

Past experiences are a resource for coping with the present

A person with dementia is no different to anyone else experiencing change: to some extent, everyone becomes anxious and looks for ways to feel reassured. Past experiences can help people to cope with the new experiences they now face. However, they can also make people think and feel differently about particular events and may mould certain views, attitudes and behaviour. A fear of the dark or a particular experience of being left alone in a darkened room might lead to a person always leaving lights switched on, for example. Memories of an unpleasant past experience can even stop a person being able to cope with the present and may make them very reluctant to change. Such feelings and behaviour apply equally to people with dementia and can explain their need to feel a sense of security, value, identity and control.

Routines and habits of a lifetime remain

Miss Greene expressed anxiety about things not being in order. What she meant may be unclear, but it is perhaps an indication that she felt a loss of control over her own affairs. Having control means having a say in how you handle your possessions, time and space. Imagine what it must be like to suddenly find yourself in a care home, when two days previously you had been living independently. Misunderstanding and confusion frequently follow moves to care homes or attendance at day centres because, to the person with dementia, the setting does not make sense. Routines of the care home such as getting up, washing, dressing, having meals, taking part in activities or going to bed can lead to increased stress, anxiety and sometimes a 'battle of wills' as they do not fit with the person's previous experiences. As far as possible, the routines of a care home or day centre should allow for individuals to follow personal choices and customs. People who previously worked on shifts, or whose job demanded early rising or who enjoyed going to bed late in the evening, may object to a routine which requires every resident to be up at 8am and expects them to be in bed by 9pm.

For people with dementia the learned habits of a lifetime are those that usually persist longest.

Whilst family and other visitors may have concerns about factors such as risk, many people with dementia have a routine and a way of coping that is unique to them. Habits and routines developed over a lifetime remain because they help create a sense of being in control.

One of the most difficult aspects of working with people with dementia is helping them to be as independent as possible – which often means **not** helping them.

The importance of relationships

Relationships are associated with those whom we choose to trust and/or who are significant to us. Our more intimate relationships with others meet our need for self-worth, love, security, respect and belonging. Relationships are a two-way process, involving a mutual meeting of needs. In all encounters with others that are significant to us, we expect to have some of these needs met. Significantly, as individuals, we choose those with whom we enter into relationships and decide how intimate they become and at what pace they get to know us.

Throughout a typical day in a home or day centre, there are many opportunities for care workers to make the person with dementia feel valued and to develop a relationship. Reminiscing and stimulating activities need not be just planned events. They can be prompted by sharing and discussing everyday matters with the person with dementia, for example:

- when accompanying the person to the dining room, stop at a window and comment on the view;
- pick up objects, such as ornaments and fruit, for the person to hold;
- encourage the person to feel the curtains, smell the flowers;
- enable the person to stroke the cat or dog (if the home allows animals).

Taking the time to find out how the person with dementia wants to be addressed can also help staff develop a better relationship. Forms of address such as 'Pop', 'Gran' or 'Dear' can be very unhelpful, especially if they have never had any children. These terms also diminish their status and can create an atmosphere in which staff do not see the people as adults. Some people will be happy for staff to use their first name; others would be offended and would prefer to be addressed formally – Mr, Mrs or Miss, for example. Always use a name for the person which is recognised and with which the individual feels comfortable.

Joining a day care group or becoming a resident of a care home may initially be an isolating experience for a person with dementia, as they are joining a ready-made group, with established friendships and levels of relationships. It can also be unnerving: 'Will they like me?' 'Will the group talk to me or will I be ignored?' 'Will I like them?' Even the most socially adept of us – and without dementia – can find it threatening. However, unlike residents, we can always choose to leave if we feel that we do not fit in. To help newcomers form a common bond with existing group members, care workers should always introduce them. A few background details about the person could be given, always ensuring that any personal information is not deemed private or confidential.

Being seen as capable

Competent functioning as an adult is based on a personal view of being seen by others to cope. We lay great emphasis on being able to cope with life's daily demands such as cooking and other household chores. Indications of being capable are:

- exercising choice;
- making the right decisions and resolving problems;
- being able to communicate;
- maintaining personal hygiene and being able to dress ourselves.

Everyone in society considers these important. However, what is 'right' or 'acceptable' or 'normal' in an individual's way of life is more problematic, as judgements are frequently based on the observer's attitudes and ideas. It is our view that determines whether people like Miss Greene are supported at home and if she is seen as capable. Our attitudes potentially present *us* with a problem.

Dementia is a shared problem

It is easy to look at a person with dementia and note what they cannot do. An individual's needs assessment will often emphasise the level of disability as opposed to the abilities the person still retains. The difficulties of remembering events, finding the right words to express feelings, or dressing in the correct order can occur because of the illness – but sometimes the difficulties are created by our responses.

People with dementia can still do things for themselves and care workers, as a result of the needs assessment, should provide opportunities for the individual to be involved in meaningful activity. This adds to their self-esteem and sense of being valued. Dependency that is created by the carers' low expectations is often related to them being too quick at completing simple tasks. One example is handing out tea with milk and sugar already added, rather than encouraging people to help themselves. Low expectations by staff can lead to a lack of opportunities for people to use their abilities and can create more difficulties later as staff cope with increasingly dependent residents or day care group members.

Providing a continuity of support

Staff should get to know the person with dementia as early as possible, so that, as the illness progresses, they can respond in a helpful way. Currently, the most usual way in a care home is to appoint a 'befriender' (sometimes called keyworker or primary care worker). It is even better if the resident can choose this person. It is important for the befriender to feel positive about the resident. A plan should be drawn up that can provide the whole team with a guide to the individual support required by each resident. This will ensure that there is a consistency and continuity in the way they are treated. It will also enable staff to avoid stereotyping.

KEY POINTS

- The routines of a care setting should allow individuals to maintain personal choices and customs.
- A person with dementia should be helped to maintain existing relationships and encouraged to make new friendships.
- Care staff should avoid creating dependency as a result of low expectations and attitudes.

EXERCISE

'Why am I being punished? Have I done something wrong?'

Cathy, the care worker, was becoming extremely frustrated with Mr Heatherington. Since coming to help him get dressed at 7.30am, he had been constantly repeating those questions over and over again, and insisting on dressing himself. It was now 8.15am and he still had not buttoned up his cardigan. How much simpler it would be just to dress Mr Heatherington but she knew that he would physically resist. Dominic, a keen trainee care worker, seemed to get on with Mr Heatherington. Cathy thought he would have more time – after all, she had all the other jobs to do. 'Dominic', she shouted.

What were Mr Heatherington's needs?

Given what is written in Chapter 1, what might Cathy have done differently?

2 Approaches to the person

Objectives:

- *To present the uniqueness of each individual and the importance of their past*
- *To identify particular approaches to understanding the person and being understood*

Allowing for difficulties

Every person is a unique individual, with physical, social, intellectual and spiritual needs. The way we strive to meet those needs, throughout our lives, moulds our individuality and uniqueness. People with dementia should also be respected as individuals, with a unique identity, personality, and life history. They have the same rights as any other adult: a right to privacy, a right to make their own decisions, a right to express feelings and a right to respect.

It can often be easier for staff to focus on what people with dementia cannot do and to have low expectations. Staff sometimes feel a sense of helplessness and respond by denying the person any opportunity to do things for themselves. This can lead to an enforced dependency, which, in turn, can lead the person to feel frustrated, angry and upset.

The changes that occur for the person with dementia do not happen all at once. The ways in which dementia affects an individual will vary from person to person. In some people, short-term memory loss is the most obvious change. In others, it is a decline in their ability to care for themselves. In others still, it is their ability to communicate, or their social graces, which decline most obviously. Some people continue to be able to carry out quite complicated actions, remember a few very fixed old memories, or keep up some previously learned habit or routine, which can lead staff to feel that they do not have dementia. Dementia does not cause loss of eyesight or hearing, although people may have poor eyesight or hearing for completely different reasons. What goes wrong is the way in which the brain makes sense of all the information it receives (see Chapter 3). Caring approaches need to take account of these changes. Given the right attitude of care workers to the help and support of the person, a degree of independence, choice and control can be maintained.

To understand and allow for these difficulties, staff should try to find out about the person's lifetime of experiences. Knowing the important memories, life experiences, routines and relationships can help them understand and see a logic for certain aspects of the person's behaviour. It can also help them to treat that person with dignity, even if the person cannot remember all their past life or has lost a sense of who they are or where they are staying. Decision-making by the person with dementia is to be encouraged, as it allows the individual to express their preference and to give consent. It can be assisted by simplifying choices at mealtimes, for example, or by taking time to listen to the person's understanding of the situation. Wherever possible, staff should avoid taking over or making assumptions based on their experience of the past choices of an individual, as these are likely to change.

Maintaining individuality and independence raises the matter of rights and risk. Sometimes a resident may choose to follow an action that poses a risk to themselves or others. It can be difficult, for example, to stop a resident who is determined to leave. However, risks can be minimised and the person's self-worth and sense of dignity can be preserved if, for example, the external layout can lead people into a safe, enclosed garden or if other diverting activities can be found en route. As with all risk, it is important to weigh up alternatives.

People with dementia from minority ethnic groups face added difficulties because of living in a country that was not necessarily their first home. During the 1930s, 1940s and 1950s, immigration into the UK by people of various ethnic origins, including Jewish, Polish and Ukrainian and those from the Indian sub-continent and Caribbean, means that individuals from these groups may now be living in care homes. Their experience may have been one of being subject to racial abuse, being in poorly paid employment, not feeling accepted, or feeling lonely and depressed. Some people may not have any close relatives in the UK, and may always have expected to return home. Some may feel that their cultural norm of being respected as an older person does not happen in this country. Similarly, others may not have learned English or, if they have learned it, reverted to their first learned language. The illness adds to their sense of isolation and feeling lost.

Responding to different realities

No two people see things in exactly the same way. Imagine that you are on a bus with a friend – you do not speak to one another during the journey but, instead, you watch and observe the changing faces and scenes through the window and have the experience of travelling with other people. At the end, you describe to each other what you saw, what you liked and did not like and how you felt on the journey. It is reasonable to assume that much of the observations, thoughts and feelings will be similar.

Differences will inevitably emerge, however, as your experience will be unique to you. Although you may have had the same journey, it is your own past experiences, mood and interests that will influence how you responded. The present reality of the experience is influenced by past factors, which are part of our 'baggage of life' experience.

Mrs Forrester is a 92-year-old resident, who has a diagnosis of dementia and has lived in a care home for two years. Most evenings she arrives in the lounge dressed in three dresses with her best cardigan on top, very agitated, and she angrily tells staff, 'I must go home at once! I have to prepare tea for Tom and Elizabeth' (her children).

What Mrs Forrester feels is genuine concern, distress and anxiety for her children. To her, the care home is not her own home. She is dressed ready to go home but strangers (staff) are trying to stop her going.

The reality for Mrs Forrester is not that of the staff. Dementia has created difficulties for her because she no longer remembers that Tom and Elizabeth are married and that she has four grandchildren. What she does remember is an experience of being a mother, which arouses feelings that influence how she responds to staff and other residents. The staff response must be to show her that she has been listened to and that her sense of worth and dignity is maintained.

Feelings matter

Residents with dementia can experience feelings of depression, worry, frustration, embarrassment or just bewilderment. Being unsure of the place that staff say is 'home', or who these strangers are called 'staff', can be extremely frustrating and bewildering. If there is no recollection of when a move happened or the reason for it, a resident may well feel distressed. Many people with dementia are so bewildered by the whole experience that they seem not to react at all; they retreat into themselves and act as if nothing unusual is happening. Staff need to react sensitively to these feelings and not dismiss them. This can help staff to understand behavioural patterns and to respond to the person with dementia in a more helpful way.

Working with the person and their reality

Despite their illness, most people with dementia can:

- remember experiences from their earlier years;
- hold opinions and views;
- offer advice;
- perform long-learned tasks and actions;
- learn new habits;
- enjoy pleasurable sensory stimuli;
- respond to and express emotions.

It becomes important, therefore, for staff to identify creative ways to bridge the gap of understanding and help the individual retain a sense of being valued.

Life story work

Life story work with people with dementia often involves assembling a dossier of personal facts or filling a scrapbook with meaningful pictures and photographs – but it is much more than that. It is a way of finding out more about who a person is. It seeks to discover what part their past life events, environments, relationships, habits, likes and dislikes have contributed to making that person a unique individual – and why they are the way they are. Life story work is a valuable opportunity for the keyworker or named staff member to collaborate with a resident in sharing their important life experiences so that a relationship and rapport is established.

It is likely that, before admission, a social worker will have written a report; this may give an outline of where the person comes from, their significant relationships and a record of their physical and mental capabilities. Some reports may include facts about the person's childhood home, their occupation and particular likes and dislikes. These give a starting point for conversation and provide important clues as to what is important for that individual.

If little information is provided, the staff member may have to take other cues, such as a person's personal mementoes, old photograph albums and family pictures, to find out the person's important and special memories. Relatives, friends and neighbours may be able to fill in any gaps. Staff must be sensitive, however, to the fact that not everyone wants other people to know all about aspects of their past history; this should be respected. Staff should also respect the different customs and beliefs of people from minority ethnic origins: for example, showing photographs of living relatives to a person with dementia of Chinese origin may cause more distress, as they associate photographs with meaning that the person has died.

Life story work can include:

- where the person was born and brought up;
- what jobs they did and with whom they worked;
- their hobbies and social interests;
- details of their significant relationships;
- family and friends;
- personal beliefs and attitudes.

Be careful not to assume that, just because a person has not married, they have not had relationships or enjoyed sexual partnerships. If a person is a lesbian or gay man, this might have been less likely to have been acknowledged or spoken about in the past.

Life story work should continue even after a person is brought in to group care: important events happening in the home or centre, such as birthdays, parties and important visitors, should all be included. By building up this picture of the whole person, their individuality and uniqueness can be seen more clearly, and staff will have greater insight and be able to respond to them more appropriately.

Reminiscence

Reminiscence is defined as 'a recollection or remembrance of some past fact or experience'. We all do it. Reminiscences are not necessarily factual accounts; they are often vivid and personal memories, which can evoke a range of emotions, from happiness and joy to anger and frustration. Reminiscing can take place at any time or any place – what is important is listening to a person's memories and valuing what is being said.

At one time, it was considered 'unhealthy' to encourage older people to remember the past, as they might dwell on previous experiences and become morbid. In recent years, however, the value of reminiscence has been recognised. By looking at the past in terms of the present, it can connect a person with their roots and help them come to terms with their current situation. Reconnecting to the past may even make the present becomes less lonely and threatening.

Reminiscence is now more widely used with people with dementia, either individually or in small groups. Confidence can be gained by focusing on what can be done and what can be remembered. The person's long-term memory is usually very strong and people with dementia often retain an ability to recall the distant past in graphic detail.

Reminiscence can increase a person's self-worth and self-esteem, when other people show an interest in their memories and also value their past lives. Reminiscence work can also be of value to carers, as the person being cared for becomes a significant individual, rather than just someone to be looked after. This can greatly improve morale and job satisfaction, and mutual respect and trust can be built up.

Multi-sensory rooms

Many homes and day care centres have set up multi-sensory rooms, sometimes called Snoezelen rooms, with bubble tubes, trailing fibre optics, twinkling and revolving lights or aromatherapy diffusers. These can provide the person with dementia with a pleasurable, sensory experience. Staff should ensure, however, that the person is not left alone in the room: the strange lights and smells can create anxiety, and people with dementia need constant reassurance. Used correctly, multi-sensory rooms can give shared, pleasurable one-to-one contact between the staff member and the person with dementia.

Music

Music can be entertaining and stimulating, and it is something that most people enjoy. Beat, rhythm, melodies and tunes do not necessarily need words to forge links with past memories and be meaningful. Music is also a therapeutic intervention to reduce anxiety and minimise behavioural problems, and can be an important aspect of care.

In many residential homes and day centres, music is frequently just a background noise from the radio or favourite records from the stereo system chosen by staff. Taste in music is individual, and the music played should reflect the different tastes of the group members. Knowing their likes and dislikes is important as, for some people, inappropriate music can create more confusion. People often respond best to songs and singers who were popular in their youth, and are not so likely to respond to current 'pop' music. However, people with dementia, like all of us, can acquire new tastes! Be prepared to experiment with music: South American rhythms, Scottish dance music, or Caribbean street band music can all lift the mood. Homes and day centres can sometimes set aside a secluded area for groups or individuals to go to listen to their favourite music.

The arts

Art and the arts cover a whole variety of activities, including music, drama, songs, poetry and creative painting. Becoming involved in any art or leisure activity can enable a person with dementia to utilise previously learned skills, perhaps learn new ones, and to express feelings and memories. For a person interested in art, the simple act of providing a brush, canvas and paints can give a freedom to be creative and to communicate in a way that does not depend on words. The painting may evoke some distant recollection for the individual and provide a discussion point for carers.

Similarly, involving a group in acting out a simple drama, comedy sketch, or song with actions, can be one way of encouraging a shared, pleasurable experience, which helps create a sense of belonging. People with dementia have an untapped potential which, if encouraged, can become important for self-expression and maintaining individuality. The only limitations are often those imposed by what care workers feel able to do: with proper support and training, there need be no limitations.

KEY POINTS

- People with dementia are unique individuals with a whole lifetime of experience behind them.
- Every person with dementia is affected by the illness in a different way.
- Care staff should be sensitive to people's differing needs, and work to maintain cultural and traditional roles.
- Care staff should identify creative ways to bridge the gap of understanding and help the individual retain a sense of being valued.
- People with dementia should be encouraged to maintain a degree of independence, however limited that might be.

EXERCISE

Mrs Morales originally moved from Spain to the UK 25 years ago. She came with her husband and family. She has begun attending day care, but is extremely upset and continually shouts, 'It's not fair – here am I, old and tired – but where are the children?'

What may be the reason for her behaving in this way?

What could be done about this?

3 What is dementia and what is not?

Objectives:

- *To explain what is happening to the brain*
- *To identify what is dementia and what is not*

Dementia is an umbrella term that describes a group of symptoms caused by the impact of disease on the brain. These symptoms include problems with memory, reasoning, understanding, learning and speech that, over a period of six months or more, are sufficient to impair the functioning of a person in their daily living. For most people, it is progressive in nature and is ultimately fatal.

Knowing whether or not a person has dementia is difficult, particularly in the early stages, as there are other illnesses, which cause the same symptoms, many of which are treatable. Also, some people rely on their social skills and habits of a lifetime to mask the impact of dementia and to cope with any loss of ability. Understanding how the brain functions and acts as the management centre of our body can help us begin to see the impact of the illness of dementia on the person.

Brain functioning

The brain is a complex organ of our body, which controls and helps us cope with the demands of living. It is a grey spongy mass, protected by the skull, and made up of billions of nerve cells that are connected to each other. It has a blood supply and is bathed in cerebral fluid. Different parts of the brain control distinct functions, although these are all interconnected in a complex way. The front part (frontal lobe) initiates our actions and then receives feedback about whether what is happening is what was intended, helping us alter our actions when necessary. The middle part (parietal lobe) helps us speak, read, move our arms and legs, and find our way around. It consists of two sides (hemispheres), one of which will be dominant: if you are right-handed, the left hemisphere will be the dominant side, and vice versa. Towards the base of the brain (brain stem) are the temporal lobes, which contain our memory bank. There is also the limbic system, which controls our intake of food and water, sleep pattern and emotions.

These different parts of the brain work together to help us cope with the different aspects of our daily functioning. The process can be likened to a factory production line. The raw materials (the stimuli) enter by different routes (eyes, ears, nose, mouth and by touch), which, through the manufacturing process, link together to produce a single article (a response). These connections in our brain are created by nerve cells linked with neurotransmitters, which pass the 'messages' (impulses) from one part of the brain to the other.

The simple act of going into a room to sit down in an armchair to talk with a resident is initiated and controlled by our brain. It demands a whole range of functions, including entering the room, looking for an armchair, seeing it, recognising it, knowing how to use it, sitting down and then remembering the social skills necessary for communication with the resident. When a person has dementia, the part (or parts) of the brain that is impaired will affect how they cope with such tasks. Damage to the temporal lobes, for example, can lead to memory impairment, usually the memory of recent things. The person may look for an armchair but only remember the one from their first home, and so not recognise where they are. Damage to the parietal lobes may lead to impaired co-ordination of movement or speech. The resident may have difficulty with spatial awareness, working out the distance between themselves and the chair. Their speech difficulties might prevent them finding the right words to express their feelings. Damage to the frontal lobe may cause residents to not recognise the consequences of going to sit in an armchair which has knitting needles left on it, for example.

Although brain function is impaired, this does not completely rob the individual of their ability to cope with the demands of daily living. There will also be marked differences in individual patterns of behaviour, depending on which part of the brain is affected.

What is dementia?

The three most common types of dementia are Alzheimer's disease, Vascular disease and Lewy Body disease.

Alzheimer's disease is the most common cause of dementia. Approximately 40 to 45 per cent of people with dementia will have Alzheimer's disease. During the course of the disease, the chemistry of the brain changes, and nerve cells and neurotransmitters are attacked. Although impairment of brain functioning is patchy at first, eventually the brain shrinks and gaps develop in the brain tissue because of these changes, which leads to an overall impairment. Alzheimer's disease is rarely hereditary, although a few people may develop the condition because of the genes they inherit.

Vascular disease leads to dementia due to damage to the blood vessels to the brain. The brain relies on a network of vessels to bring it oxygen-bearing blood. If the oxygen supply to the brain fails, brain cells are likely to die. Symptoms of vascular disease can either happen suddenly, perhaps following a stroke, or over a period of time due to heart disease or hypertension. Smoking and lack of exercise can be contributory factors. Around 25 to 30 per cent of people with dementia will have vascular disease. It is more common in men due to the higher risk factors of heart disease. The person affected may experience some difficulties with short-term memory and communication: speech often becomes slurred, and there may be a slight paralysis of one side of the body. People with vascular disease may also have some insight into their own condition and this may lead to depression or mood swings.

Lewy Body disease gets its name from the tiny, spherical structures made of proteins that develop inside the nerve cells. Their presence in the brain leads to the degeneration and death of the brain tissue affecting memory, concentration and language skills. Individuals may experience visual hallucinations and also develop physical problems such as slowness of movement, stiffness and tremor. Around 20 per cent of people with dementia will have Lewy Body disease. People with this form of dementia seem to have an excessive sensitivity and react adversely to particular types of medication used to treat other illnesses and behavioural difficulties.

Other forms of dementia

Less common forms of dementia are caused by degenerative conditions, infection and the effect of toxins on the brain. It is also increasingly being recognised that people who have had a head injury (Acquired Brain Injury), through an accident involving loss of consciousness, may be more likely to develop dementia.

Parkinson's disease, Huntington's disease, Down's syndrome and **Pick's disease** are examples of degenerative conditions where symptoms of dementia can become apparent. People with **Parkinson's disease** will experience short-term memory impairment, poor concentration, slowness of thinking, indecisiveness and apathy. People born with **Huntington's disease** may be in their 30s or 40s when the symptoms of dementia develop. This can lead to feelings of depression and paranoid ideas, although the person retains a recognition of family and friends. People with **Down's syndrome** are more likely to develop Alzheimer's disease because of their chromosomal defect. In **Pick's disease**, people's personality and behaviour are initially more affected than memory because damage to the brain cells is more localised in the frontal lobe.

Infections of the brain include **CJD** (Creutzfeldt-Jakob disease) and **AIDS** (Acquired Immune Deficiency Syndrome). CJD is caused by infectious agents called prions, which attack brain tissue. The variant form (vCJD) has been linked to BSE (Bovine Spongiform Encephalopathy), a prion disease affecting cattle, although the number of people with vCJD is low. People with **AIDS HIV** (Human Immunodeficiency Virus) can also develop dementia in the later stages of their illness.

Korsakoff's syndrome can be described as a toxic dementia, as chronic alcohol dependence over many years can lead to memory loss and damage to the frontal lobe of the brain. There is evidence to suggest that, if a person lessens their consumption of alcohol, the dementia may stabilise, although existing brain damage will remain.

These different types of dementia are termed 'irreversible', as there is no means, at present, of regenerating nerve cells. However, Vascular disease might be prevented by not smoking, having a healthier diet and more exercise. Similarly, Korsakoff's syndrome might be prevented by not becoming chronically dependent on alcohol.

The impact of dementia on the individual

Dementia predominantly affects older people, particularly those aged 60 and over, but it is not due to the ageing process. The impact of dementia on each individual will be different. Some individuals may have short-term memory problems but no communication difficulty at the beginning, whilst others may have both. Some early signs of dementia are:

Memory impairment
Initially short-term memory is affected: the person may forget where they have put things, the names of family and friends, or where they live. They have increasing difficulty in learning new information. Long-term memories of the past remain strongest and often lead to things being said now as if they have just occurred, when, in fact, they happened many years ago.

Aphasia (difficulty in finding the right words to express thoughts and feelings)
Speech using the right words can be adversely affected. Crucial to communication is responding to the person's feelings. Recognising cues that relate to the person can help understand their needs and assist meaningful interaction. If speech difficulties exist, other means of communication, such as singing, poetry, writing or art, can help the person relate to others.

Apraxia (impaired ability to carry out motor activities despite intact motor function)
Tasks such as tying shoelaces, getting dressed or making a cup of tea correctly can become increasingly difficult for the person with dementia. They may know what to do but they cannot put the actions together in the correct order or are unable to know where they should begin and so sit helplessly. There is nothing wrong with the physical movement of their arms and legs but they are unable to process their thinking into actions. Sensitive prompting by staff can help remind the person of each step they need to take.

Agnosia (failure to recognise significant people or identify objects despite intact sensory function)
We depend a great deal on our vision and our ability to interpret what we see to enable us to cope with daily living. People with dementia have an inability to translate the information from what they see with their eyes into a correct response. This means that, if asked to pick up a spoon, the person may look straight at it, yet fail to recognise the object as a spoon. However, place the spoon in the person's hands and the feel of the spoon can prompt the memory of how to use it correctly. This inability to recognise objects can extend to people, even those who have been most closely associated with them. Also, when the person with dementia looks into a mirror, they do not see an image of themselves but a stranger staring back at them.

Medication for dementia

There is no cure for dementia. Current new drug treatments act to halt the speed of progression of Alzheimer's disease for those in the early stages of the illness. If prescribed early, the person appears to show improvement in behaviour and function for a time. It is essential that people prescribed the current drugs (trade names include Aricept, Exelon and Reminyl) must comply rigidly with the medication regime.

Dementia – the later stages

In the later stages, there is a more global impairment of brain functioning. The person may lose control of many physical functions, including bladder control, becoming incontinent by night and day. Bowel problems may occur, including constipation or diarrhoea, and some people may be faecally incontinent.

Weight loss is a common feature for people with dementia, and eating difficulties such as poor co-ordination when swallowing can occur in the later stages of the illness. However, it may also be due to the mechanisms in the brain that control appetite and weight maintenance having been damaged by the dementia. This explains why people may eat well, or even overeat to the extent of eating anything, even plants or paper that are lying around, but still lose weight. This part of the brain also controls the internal body clock, and sleep can become disturbed, if it is damaged. The individual may sleep for longer or shorter periods than usual and may be awake during the night but asleep during the day. Although dementia is usually fatal after seven to nine years, some people can live longer than this.

Dementia creates perplexing problems for staff. Sometimes the combination of the affects of the illness with their past routines and lifestyle leads to apparently contradictory actions and behaviour. Understanding the consequences of dementia for the person can help staff ensure that their expectations of individuals are realistic and efforts accurately directed. Good care depends on the carer considering the person – and seeing if there is a reason for changes or difficult behaviour – and endeavouring to meet their needs. Staff should consider whether they could be more tolerant of a person's behaviour. Sometimes problems are only temporary.

What is not dementia?

The diagnosis and detection of dementia presents difficulties for doctors, as other physical illnesses, depression and acute confusion can mimic the symptoms of dementia. The difference is that these can usually be treated. If a resident suddenly becomes more disorientated, has increasing memory difficulty and communication problems, it should not be assumed that their dementia has got worse. A first course of action should always be to ask the resident's GP to make a clinical assessment and diagnosis. It may be necessary for a referral to the specialist consultant in a hospital, where more extensive diagnostic tests can be carried out.

Physical illness

Although people with dementia may not be able to say if they are feeling unwell or describe where they are feeling pain, it should never be assumed that an increased level of disorientation or memory problems are a result of the progress of dementia. Chest infections, thyroid problems, heart trouble, poor diet, change of medication, vitamin B_{12} deficiency and being stressed can lead to signs of dementia. Once recognised, and with appropriate treatment, the person can show improvement. Carers have to keep a special lookout for signs of a sudden deterioration in a person with dementia, which may mean that there is a physical illness or mental condition as well as the dementia.

Depression

Depression is a common condition in older people and it can also occur in people with dementia, although it is not necessarily caused by the illness. Common symptoms include:

- poor concentration and forgetfulness;
- lack of emotional response (or constant crying);
- lack of motivation and a declining interest in daily living;
- poor sleep and loss of appetite (or the complete opposite);
- mood disturbance, often more marked in the morning.

Depression often comes on slowly over a number of weeks. Speech, thought and movement can be slowed but, as the day progresses, the person becomes more alert and orientated. People with dementia who have depression frequently respond to antidepressant medication, although it may have to be continued over a long period of time.

Acute confusion

Acute confusion is caused by direct damage to the brain due to injury or disease, general illnesses, which disturb brain functioning, or poisons and drugs, which affect the brain. It often appears very quickly and may be brief in duration. Causes can include:

- pneumonia;
- heart condition;
- constipation;
- urinary or bowel infection;
- the side effects of some prescribed drug medication.

This sometimes means that the person has spells when they are alert and other times when they are unaware of where they are. They may become much more muddled or disorientated and even begin to see things – hallucinations – which are not there in reality. The person may become much more fearful, irritable or aggressive. Once the underlying cause is discovered, treatment should lead to a return to the previous state of health.

Staff who work in day or residential care are often well placed to observe changes in the person's mood and thinking, and their ability to carry out day to day activities. When staff feel that depression or acute confusion is affecting a person, this should be recorded in writing and brought to the attention of the manager or supervisor. It should not be assumed that the dementia has got worse. The changes noted can then be drawn to the attention of the visiting doctor, community psychiatric nurse (CPN) or nurse. If symptoms appear quickly, it is likely that a physical illness may be the cause of a sudden change in the person's wellbeing. The illnesses mentioned in this section are treatable with medication and the person can return to their previous level of functioning.

The side effects of medication

Changes in a person's behaviour and mood can also be a result of prescribed medication. Wrong or too high drug medication can often make the person sleepy throughout the day and more confused at night, and may cause aggressive, hostile and more disturbed behaviour. The person may fall more easily. It can lead to development of tremors, loss of appetite, and jerky movements if the medication continues over a long period of time. Staff should continually be alert to this and avoid using other medication, such as sedatives, to reduce behavioural problems. Sedatives are rarely appropriate for people with dementia, although exceptions might be made when the resident's behaviour poses a serious risk to themselves or others. However, they should only be given as a last resort, when all other approaches have been exhausted.

KEY POINTS

- It is usually short-term memory that is lost first, although dementia can affect all the brain's functions, and is ultimately fatal.
- Alzheimer's disease usually presents gradually and slowly, sometimes with almost imperceptible change.
- In Lewy Body disease, there are marked swings and fluctuations in symptoms. Visual hallucinations are a prominent feature of the disease.
- In Vascular disease, there may be a long spell when nothing changes and then, abruptly, there will be quite a marked change in thinking, physical functions and self-care ability.
- There is no cure for dementia although current drug treatments for Alzheimer's disease can reduce the speed of progression of the illness.
- Sudden, abrupt swings in mood, changes of behaviour, and short periods of impairment in the person's ability to perform activities of daily life may be caused by treatable conditions.

QUIZ

Try this quiz with your colleagues:

1 Which is the most common type of dementia?

2 Is there any known cure for dementia?

3 Which organ of the body is most affected by dementia?

4 Is it easy to diagnose someone with dementia?

5 Does a sudden change in behaviour mean the person has dementia?

6 Why are acute confusion and depression not like dementia?

7 I sometimes forget things. Do I have dementia?

8 Is the use of medication a good idea to cope with difficult behaviour?

(See suggested answers in Appendix 2 on page 101)

4 Health matters

Objectives:

- *To stress the importance of accurate diagnosis and assessment, and the role of the doctor in attending to people with dementia*
- *To raise staff awareness of physical health issues*

The importance of accurate diagnosis and assessment

In the early stages of dementia, a firm diagnosis can be difficult because, as mentioned in the previous chapter, treatable conditions such as depression, urinary tract infection and other illnesses can also cause impairment of memory, communication and understanding. Consequently, the family doctor should carry out a medical examination and do an assessment of the person's physical, psychological and functional capabilities. Discussion with the person and their carer and/or family can also help establish how that person's current functioning ability differs from before. Accurate early diagnosis is crucial so that treatable illnesses can be dealt with, leading to an improvement in the person's wellbeing and capacity to fulfil activities of daily living. Early identification of Alzheimer's disease is also important, as there are new drug treatments that can reduce the speed of progression and help maintain the person's ability to function.

For the individual, an early diagnosis would give them the chance to undertake advance planning of their own finances, attend to other important personal matters, and express a preference in treatment. It also allows a discussion with doctors, nurses and carers about what support is required. It is important that information about a diagnosis of dementia is shared with the person and their relatives. However, the process of advising the person with dementia and informing them of their condition can be extremely stressful for those who are able to understand the significance of their condition. A sensitive approach is required, and, ideally, an ongoing relationship with the person to provide follow-up support.

For those living in care homes or attending day care without a *definite* diagnosis of dementia, staff should be alert to detecting any changes in the person's memory, reasoning, concentration and daily living skills. Such changes should be brought to the attention of senior staff, the visiting nurse or doctor, or relatives.

As dementia progresses, so needs change; good care involves procedures for regular, individualised assessment and care planning. The review of care plans is done most effectively by those who have a significant relationship with the person. Review discussions should involve the keyworker, as well as other professionals, such as the doctor, social worker or community nurse. When appropriate, a family member may be invited. Reviews should ideally occur on a three-monthly basis, so that, when needs change, other more specialist assessments can be introduced as necessary.

The doctor's role in attending to people with dementia

In the care home – and often in a day centre – the family doctor has an important role in providing staff with a medical assessment of the person with dementia. This assessment should be followed up regularly. In providing continuing care for people with dementia, changing needs require constant monitoring and review, and specific health issues common to the people with dementia noted. Doctors should, if possible, be involved in helping staff develop the individualised care plan for the person with dementia.

As the doctor retains responsibility for the individual's day-to-day general health and wellbeing, staff also need to make the doctor aware of any physical and mental changes in the person. Dementia is frequently not the cause of changes in health. The doctor is also the gatekeeper to other services that may be required, such as a consultant psychiatrist or a geriatrician, or further investigation in hospital.

Promoting a healthy lifestyle

Whilst some of the health problems experienced by people with dementia can be those commonly associated with growing older, they can also be a consequence of their own chosen lifestyle and even of living in a group care setting. The duty of care that staff have to look after residents with dementia and attend to their physical wellbeing brings into sharp focus, and sometimes conflict, the balance between promoting a healthy lifestyle and allowing the individual to maintain their habits and preferences of a lifetime. Care plans need to record these preferences to ensure that there is a balance between individual choice and the routines of the care home, and between an individual taking personal risks and jeopardising the health and safety of other residents and staff.

Diets and menu planning

Care home staff can face situations in which some residents experience problems of obesity and constipation due to the combination of regular meals and reduced levels of activity, whilst other residents lose weight for no apparent reason. Constipation may be a result of diets being low in roughage (fibre) or the side effects of medication. It can cause distress, restlessness, sleeplessness and pain for individuals, as well as increased confusion. A local dietician may be able to help with planning a menu, in which the fibre, vitamin, protein and fat content of the meals have been accurately measured. The provision of a variety of drinks and sufficient fluids is also important.

For those who lose weight, there can be a variety of reasons. It may be a result of their constant activity around the home or eating difficulties caused by ill-fitting dentures, or painful gums or teeth. It may also be a result of having particular food likes and dislikes, which are not being catered for, or not being able to sit and eat at the dining table for any length of time.

Any dramatic and sudden change in diet or appetite may indicate a change in physical health and should not be assumed to be a consequence of the dementia.

Alcohol intake

Many people with dementia will continue to enjoy a drink – or may even start to drink – either on a daily basis or on special occasions such as Christmas, birthdays or social events. Staff may need to watch the amount consumed, however, as short-term memory impairment may lead to the person forgetting that they have had a drink. Nevertheless, a person has a right to drink if they so wish, and a staff team whose care plan attempts to restrict when and how much is consumed may encounter difficult, angry, unco-operative, disruptive behaviour until that person obtains a drink. Consequently, when devising a care plan, careful consideration needs to be given to the effects of restricting alcohol on that person and on other residents and staff.

For those who have developed Korsakoff's Syndrome as a result of chronic alcoholism, a major reduction in alcoholic consumption can lead to an improvement in memory and physical health. In all situations, if a person is on regular medication, a check should be made with the doctor to find out if alcohol is permitted.

Smoking

Smoking can sometimes play a part in the development of Vascular disease. It is also incriminated in the cause of other conditions, including lung cancer and heart disease. Nevertheless, as with drinking, a person has a right to smoke if they so wish, and to attempt to stop that person may create other difficulties. However, as well as health problems, there are also safety hazards associated with smoking: for example, people with dementia who smoke may forget to extinguish their cigarette and so potentially cause a fire. Some supervision may be necessary, therefore, to avoid unacceptable risks to themselves and to other residents. As the dangers of passive smoking are increasingly recognised and acknowledged, it might be beneficial to set aside specific rooms or areas for smoking – or no-smoking areas, depending on the percentage of residents who smoke.

Incontinence

People with dementia can suffer from incontinence, although it is more common for people in the later stages of the illness. There are many simple causes, however, which can often be treated, and it should not be assumed that because a person is incontinent they need remain so. Incontinence may be due to diuretic medication given at the wrong dose or at the wrong time, urinary infections, constipation or prostatism in men.

For some people with dementia, there is a loss of awareness that they need to pass water or faeces. Equally, they may no longer recognise where the toilet is and may accidentally soil themselves or empty their bowels somewhere other than the toilet. These actions have to be recognised for what they are – symptoms of the illness – not deliberate, offensive actions. With appropriate intervention, this behaviour can often be altered and contained. Clearly marked toilets and attention to food and fluid intake can help these problems. Understanding why the person is behaving in a particular way can help staff cope with seemingly difficult behaviour.

Vision and hearing

Loss of sharpness of vision and a reduction in the range of hearing is common for older people as part of normal ageing. For the person with dementia, visual and hearing impairment can be even more incapacitating, as they contribute to increased confusion or awkward behaviour. With these faculties improved, behaviour often settles. Regular tests should be made to determine whether there are sight or hearing problems. Hearing aids, when worn, need to be fitted properly and switched on, remembering that hearing aids amplify all sound and can be extremely distressing in a noisy day centre or sitting room. Similarly, spectacles need to be clean and worn correctly.

Falls

Falls are common in older people. However, those with dementia may experience more than most because of the effects of their illness, which can cause loss of spatial awareness and co-ordination, problems with walking and a lack of awareness of safety and self-protection. It should also be remembered that other factors can add to the likelihood of falls, such as poor eyesight, poorly fitting shoes and other foot problems, badly placed furniture, unclearly marked steps, failure to use walking sticks, and poor supervision. Regular health check-ups for the person with dementia, as well as regular reviews of health and safety features of the home or day care centre, can minimise most of these additional risks.

Depression

Staff should always be looking out for signs of depression in the person with dementia. Signs include obvious sadness, irritability and agitation, if they are slower than usual in their actions, have little interest, or poor concentration, with symptoms worse in the morning. Also if their sleeping pattern is disturbed or if they wake up very early. Depression is a treatable condition and antidepressant medication can often be beneficial.

Giving out medication

People with dementia frequently forget to take medication because they do not feel unwell. They may need reminding, or medicines may have to be dispensed by the carer. Staff should keep a record of those people who have difficulty swallowing tablets or who dislike the taste, and agree appropriate action. Ethically and legally, the medication should not be given without the person's permission, by hiding it or disguising it in food or drink, for example. A person has the right to refuse the medication. If consent is given, staff should check whether tablets can be crushed or whether they are a slow release that requires them to be taken whole. Some medication is also available in a liquid form, with a sweet, pleasant taste, which may be easier for staff to administer and for people to swallow. Medication times and the compliance with dosage instructions are crucial and the local authority's Registration and Quality Assurance Teams will expect there to be a clear procedure for the giving out and recording of medications over a 24-hour period. All medicines have potential side effects and staff should be aware of the effects of changing medication, failure to comply with dosage instructions and the effects of a combination of medicines. If there is an obvious change in the person's behaviour or state of health, staff should contact the senior member of staff or call the doctor.

Medication to control behaviour

Nowadays, doctors should not prescribe a drug for disturbed behaviour without a proper medical and psychological assessment of the person with dementia. Giving any medication as a response to difficult behaviour should only be regarded as a last resort, when other non-drug interventions and approaches have been tried. Sleeping tablets and sedatives, which are given to reduce agitation and behavioural problems, frequently create more problems. The individual may be very drowsy and sleepy during the day and night due to over-sedation but not necessarily sleep well at night. Few medicines are free from unwanted side effects. Antidepressant tablets, which are very effective in treating depression in older people and in people with dementia, have side effects such as low blood pressure, constipation and confusion.

Neuroleptics (anti-psychotic drugs) are used to manage hallucinations and delusion, and are also used in managing behaviour. These drugs adversely affect older people and are associated with causing the following side effects:

- slowness and difficulty initiating movement;
- an inability to sit still or stay in same place;
- involuntary, repeated or abnormal movements of muscles of the mouth, arms and legs, or body.

These side effects can lead staff to think that the symptoms are caused by the person's underlying dementia. Treatment with neuroleptic drugs, if used, should begin with the lowest possible dose and be constantly reviewed. The risks, as well as any benefits, should always be considered. For people with Lewy Body disease, who are still being prescribed medication, there is a greater risk of exacerbating the symptoms of the illness.

If drugs are prescribed, their effectiveness is likely to be only in the short term. The care of such individuals involves doctors, nurses and staff, and it is important for everyone working in care homes and day care centres to remember that these patients often cannot complain properly. Investigation can be quite easy and treatment may be effective. Some of the problems are not just the problems of the person, but can be a result of the attitudes and responses of those around them.

KEY POINTS

- Regular assessments should be carried out.
- There should be a clear care plan for staff to follow.
- All medication has potential side effects for the person with dementia.
- Whilst promoting a healthy lifestyle, staff should allow the individual to maintain their habits and preferences of a lifetime.
- There should be a good balanced diet with regular activity.
- Problems of incontinence should not be seen as an inevitable part of dementia.
- Sudden changes in the person's wellbeing should be referred for a medical check.

EXERCISE

Mrs Braithwaite, who has just been diagnosed with dementia, is a quiet, 80-year-old widow, who takes pride in her appearance. She attends day care, where her normal routine is to help staff set the tables for lunch. Today she has arrived very unkempt, wearing old clothes, with a bruise to her forehead, and smelling strongly of urine. In talking to her, staff find that she seems very anxious and unsure about where she is. She refuses to help and becomes extremely angry, and physically resists any help from staff.

Why might she be like this?

5 Behaviour as a response to the living environment

Objective:

- *To encourage recognition that behaviour can be a response to the living environment*

The behaviour of people with dementia is frequently a response to the internal, physical layout and design of the care home or day care centre. This is because the impairment of their short-term memory and perception makes it more difficult for them to remember where they are in a building and to make sense of their immediate environment. Interpreting the reasons why a resident enters other residents' bedrooms, or continually gets angry when trying to find their way to the toilet or dining room, or is upset and crying because they want to go home, requires patience and understanding. What might be regarded as difficult behaviour may simply be that person's way of expressing frustration at getting lost or being in unfamiliar surroundings, or feeling insecure and unsettled. Such feelings are not always helped by the standardised layout of many homes, in which all the bedroom doors are of the same wood veneer, long corridors are painted in bland colour schemes, and there is a lack of understandable signs indicating the toilet or dining room.

Whatever the explanation, a person's behaviour is usually a valid response to the world as experienced by that person. The danger is always that our personal views and attitudes can lead us to ignore the impact of the internal built environment and lay the problem on the resident. The size of the building, and whether it is newly built for 60 residents or an older property for 20 residents, are key factors in understanding the reasons for people's behaviour. This chapter aims to encourage a greater awareness of the impact of the built environment on the behaviour of the person with dementia and how staff can make changes and creative modifications to help people adapt.

There are five important principles to be considered, based on a general agreement of opinion from research and from people working in the specialist care of people with dementia. Buildings should:

- make sense;
- help way finding (enabling people to find their way around);
- provide a therapeutic environment;
- provide a safe environment;
- minimise staff stress.

A building should make sense

For most people with dementia, their strongest memories will be of their own home, perhaps their very first home as a child. It should not be surprising, therefore, if a new resident of a large, 60-bed care home becomes anxious and agitated as they search unsuccessfully for the bedroom they remember from their past. In trying to make sense of the unfamiliar surroundings of the care home, the individual may believe they are in a hotel, hospital or workplace, and their behaviour may reflect this. Consequently, the internal layout of the home should help residents to see what is familiar from their life experience, prompt them to go where they need to go and help create a domestic, homely, living environment.

The overall décor of the home – the wallpaper, carpets, curtains and light fittings – could all be reminiscent of the 1930s, 1940s or 1950s, which is the most familiar period for the current generation of residents. Carpets in public areas and corridors can help create a quieter, more homely atmosphere and a feeling of warmth. It is important to have sufficient lighting but, as the bright fluorescent lighting in many homes creates a harshness and an institutional feel, other softer lighting such as table lamps could also be used.

Lounges and sitting rooms should be inviting places to sit and relax. Using an assortment of traditional, old-fashioned chairs, perhaps also reminiscent of an earlier period, can be particularly beneficial for people with dementia as they can make them feel more at home. Having an assortment of chairs and the odd sofa, perhaps donated by the resident's relatives, can also be beneficial, as they are more recognisable and can lessen a person's confusion if the furniture is not all the same design. A fireplace, once a standard feature of most homes, can provide a homely focus for the room, with chairs placed in a semi-circle around it.

Making corridors look like streets or landings may sometimes be more useful than making them homely, because houses and flats rarely have corridors in them. Managers of a home in Glasgow decided to paint the corridor to look like an entrance to an old-fashioned tenement. The walls were painted in a similar colour to how the tenement would have been, and the bedroom doors were made to look like flat doors and painted in bright colours with a brass door-knocker, brass number and brass nameplate. They report that this made sense to many of the residents and helped reduce agitation.

A building should help way finding

The internal layout of a care home or day centre can create a dependency by people with dementia on staff to help them find their way to the bedroom, public rooms or toilet. As a result, the person loses their independence and coping skills, as staff feel it necessary to spend time escorting the resident. This may lead to a loss of dignity, embarrassment and even anger for the resident, particularly if they wanted to go to the toilet but could not see it, or the care worker did not arrive in time. Residents can be helped to find their way with good landmarks (pictures and objects, for example) and good signage.

Toilets

Toilets are the most important place to find. Unfortunately, many buildings make this difficult because:

- toilets are out of sight of the living areas;
- most door signs are too high and too modern.

Some older people, as part of the ageing process, will develop a stoop in their posture, which means that their level of vision is lower than it was before. Even when standing by the toilet door, some people would be unable to see a sign at normal height. A person with dementia may have the additional problem of being unable to understand either the word 'toilet' or the modern matchstick–people symbols.

The answer to the toilet door problem is to make it more obvious and different from other doors in the building. Some homes put up signs, with both words, such as toilet/WC/lavatory, and pictures, such as a picture of an old-style cistern and pan on the door. The words and pictures should be meaningful to the residents, and placed at their eye level. It may not be attractive to have a picture of a toilet on the door but, before finally deciding, watch the residents to see whether it works: it may be worthwhile if it gives them some independence.

Colours can also help if they are very contrasting and bright: although the ability to tell one colour from another can diminish with age, it often remains best in the red/yellow area of the spectrum. Pater Noster Nursing Home in Waltham Abbey, Essex, painted their toilet door-frame red, hung an object beside the door and put a sign on the door. This was very helpful for residents. Other homes have used yellow or bright orange. All of the homes with colours and signs report that this has enabled some of the residents to find their own way.

Bedrooms

Bedrooms are another key place for residents but few homes have any guide to finding them. All the doors look the same, except for a number or sometimes a small nameplate. There are a variety of ways to help people with dementia find their own rooms. For example, some will remember a number, be able to read their name, or recognise their photograph or picture of a favourite place or hobby, whilst others need a solid object such as a plant or a door-knocker.

Remember that residents are individuals and no one system will help all of them. The answer is to try different ideas. It can even be useful to have several cues, such as name, number, photograph and door-knocker, so that residents can manage at least one of them.

For those with en-suite toilet facilities in the bedroom, many of these sign, symbol and colour combinations can be used to help residents recognise the toilet/bathroom.

Communal areas

Many communal rooms, such as lounges and dining rooms, are behind closed doors and, even when the doors are open, give little indication about what goes on in the room so that the resident is prepared. For example, whilst some residential homes have a separate dining room, others simply have tables in multi-purpose rooms with no indication of what happens there or when. Residents may have their meals at a table that earlier had been used for craft work or games. This situation adds to the disorientation of a person with dementia, and staff should make a conscious effort to provide cues, such tablecloths and salt and pepper pots, to help them.

Some ideas to consider are:

- Living area doors should have panels of glass in them so that residents can see what the room is. This can be done whether adapting an existing building or building a new one.
- Careful positioning of plants, pictures and hangings to make it easier for people to recognise certain corridors, hallways and dining rooms.
- Good lighting is vital in helping residents to find their way round the home. Related to this is the importance of having flooring, which is non-reflecting: people with dementia often think that shiny floors are pools of water and are fearful of walking on them.

A design challenge when planning a specialist area for people with dementia is to make all doors visible from everywhere within that area, so that, wherever the resident is, they can see where they want to be. Toilets, in particular, ought to be visible from the sitting room or lounge.

A building should provide a therapeutic environment

A therapeutic environment is one that is relaxing and stress reducing, and enables the person with dementia to engage in meaningful activity and function as well as they are able. It should reduce the uncertainty and fear that are the disabling consequences of dementia. A therapeutic environment is one that provides:

- *Opportunities for purposeful activity*
Some residents like to continue with household chores such as washing up and preparing snacks. Wherever possible, they should have access to a kitchen, or kitchen area. Mountview Home in Callander simply has a sink in the corner of the sitting room, which is used by residents to wash up and then put away the china. Such familiar chores can lessen anxiety and encourage communication. Other ideas that can help keep some people happily busy are a garden with a greenhouse, a conservatory with plants to water or raised flowerbeds, or a domestic-scale laundry and washing line.

- *The right level of stimulation*
Too much noise and busyness in a home at one time can create disorientation and cause residents to behave in more agitated ways. Staff should aim for a quiet environment with only meaningful noise, and avoid having televisions left on all day or the continual sound of music from their favourite radio station playing in the public areas.

Being able to sit and watch, without having to respond, is an activity enjoyed by many people with dementia. A large foyer and low window sills with a view are much appreciated. Activities such as games and crafts are also important and there should be space where these can take place.

An attractive, welcoming and sweet-smelling bathroom can provide opportunities for a good sensory experience and quiet relaxation. Some residents can be resistant to bath times because of the stark unfamiliarity of the bathroom, which is often used by staff for additional storage space. It is not difficult to improve many bathrooms with more domestic décor, removing the boxes of incontinence pads that are often stored in the corner, and moving any aids, such as hoists, into cupboards when not being used.

● *Reminders to residents about their individual identity*
Residents with dementia need constant reminding about who they are. Single rooms provided unfurnished are the best way of achieving this because the room is then likely to be full of the resident's own possessions. In Dalwhinny Lodge Care Home in Peebles, the staff adapted a room to be a 1930s café. The relatives helped by providing memorabilia. It now provides a familiar place for residents to take a cup of tea or coffee. Such ideas help people with dementia reminisce and remember their previous life experiences.

Buildings should provide a safe environment

Providing a safe environment is often translated by staff as meaning that they cannot allow risk. This is often brought into sharp focus by the resident, who is unable to understand the consequences of their own actions, and goes walking about alone. However, we should not expect that a person with dementia would want to remain seated all day long. There will be occasions when they will want to go for a walk outside, be naturally inquisitive about something, actively take exercise or try to follow some long-learned routine. Other residents will continually pace up and down the same corridor or round and round the building.

The staff team then have to balance the fact that no group care environment is without risk and decide how they allow residents the right level of independence and freedom to walk about. A feeling of being confined can sometimes make individuals try hard to escape, so providing plenty of space and lots of diverting activities can help give the person the opportunity to stop and do something else.

Indoors

Concealed plugs, safety radiators and thermostatic controls on hot water are now customary in most homes. They are especially important for people with dementia who usually have impaired reasoning. For safety and security reasons, some homes attempt to conceal doors that they do not want the residents to enter by 'painting them out' and making them the same colour as the wall. However, some residents might be further confused by seeing staff entering and leaving an apparent wall, so this may not always be sensible. Cupboards or plants may be a better way of concealing a door. When planning new buildings, doors that are not for residents' access should be 'hidden', as far as possible.

Fire regulations can pose problems. Invariably, fire doors are at the end of corridors. As the door is so prominent, the person with dementia is drawn to it and discovers that they can easily open it and get through, which may create difficulties for both residents and staff. Fire doors can be made less obviously a door and more like a window in some cases, although a clear exit sign is essential. If designing from scratch, you will be able to locate them in rooms in such a way that they are not in a direct line of vision of the residents.

Increasingly, some homes are adapting the standard 'pull cord' nurse call systems and connecting passive alarms, pressure pads and movement detectors, which are activated at times when the resident is alone or considered at risk. More sophisticated systems are linked to computers that are programmed to suit each resident's routine. Whilst they are an aid to staff, they do not replace the important face-to-face contact that residents have with staff.

Outdoors

Providing a safe outdoor space can be very important for active residents, and, rather than attempt to restrict or confine the person, the space can be designed so that it is not an invitation to leave. For example, a straight path to a gate, to the visitors' car park or onto a main road will lead disorientated people clearly in that direction. A winding path should take them past something that will distract them. Some homes have designed a path that takes residents from one door of a sitting room around the building to a door on the other side. Other homes have discovered that residents do not walk off the path if there is border of flowers and shrubs alongside the path. Gardens, raised flowerbeds and garden tubs should focus people's attention inwards. Certain plants can encourage sensory stimulation, such as those with a strong, sweet perfume, with soft or feathery leaves, interesting shapes and vibrant colours. Thickly planted shrubs can also help obscure and soften the impact of what may be seen as a restricting fence or wall.

A building should minimise stress for staff

Face-to-face care for people with dementia is incredibly draining. The work can demand a level of emotional input and a degree of personal energy that is utterly exhausting. Staff must have somewhere to go, where they can laugh or cry or just be private. It must be in a part of the home away from the residents. Staff need to feel valued and be fully participating in the life of the home when they are there, but also given space and time whilst on shift to go away and recharge their energy levels. Such spaces need to be found, adapted or created, either within an existing building or a new one.

KEY POINTS

- Buildings should be as homely as possible and make sense to the person with dementia.
- Given the right cues, residents with dementia may be able to find their way round.
- An environment should provide opportunities for relaxation, as well as purposeful activity.
- A safe environment should be created, whilst allowing residents the freedom to move around and take exercise.
- Staff should have their own, separate space.

EXERCISE

Discuss with colleagues how, by having £50 to spend in the home, you might help way finding, or make it more homely.

6 Behaviour as a response to the daily routine

Objectives:

- *To recognise that behaviour can be a response to daily routine*
- *To encourage recognition that behaviour can be a response to the attitude and approach of staff and other people in their environment*

A typical day in any home will involve set routines such as getting up, washing, dressing, having meals and going to bed. These routines, although necessary, should allow for residents to have their own choices and customs. It is not unusual for people, whose job demanded early rising or who previously did shift work, to be up and about at the crack of dawn or, alternatively, later in the morning. For people with dementia, these learned habits of a lifetime may be those that persist longest and are therefore important to tolerate. Although people spend less time in day care centres, there are often still routines that need to be observed, and customs and patterns of behaviour which are important to recognise and accept from people with dementia.

Mrs Begum is a Moslem lady, who has prayed five times each day all her life. To give her life familiar structure as her dementia progresses, she will need help to continue with these learned routines. Understanding the reasons for her behaviour and having a consistent response should be the focus of a care plan.

A care plan should be a working document and not something that is drawn up once and never looked at again. As the care needs change, the individual plans should be reviewed and updated. A care plan helps staff maintain a consistency and continuity of support, which can help the individual feel less anxious and insecure. By setting objectives for the support of each individual, the care team can readily identify how they are doing.

The most effective care plans are generally produced when all the staff team has been involved in discussion of the individual's needs. Effective care plans:

- require regular review and adjustment, according to the changing needs and behaviour of the person;
- agree on how minimum disruption can be caused to the preferred routines and choices of the person;
- focus on encouraging the person's retained skills and strengths;
- tailor the support so as not to create dependency by taking over tasks that the person is still able to do with gentle prompting;
- help staff respond appropriately to certain behaviours.

Being responsive to changing needs requires a culture of good written and verbal communication. A system of record keeping is needed, which allows ease of access for all staff to refer to the care plan and to write up changes. Time for discussion between staff of different shifts allows for a sharing of ideas and views. It can support those under pressure and help develop a consistent, agreed course of action, particularly when difficulties arise that create staff stress. Discussions that involve relatives and the person with dementia are also useful in identifying and formulating the care plan. If this is not wholly feasible, then family, friends or an advocate might be consulted to ensure that the person has a voice. In devising a care plan, consideration should be given to the overall wellbeing of the person.

Wellbeing

Feeling that 'all is well' in our lives is related to not being ill and to our sense of self-worth: being in meaningful relationships, being able to trust other people, having a sense of achievement and being able to express our individuality. In other words, we need to know that we matter. So do people with dementia: they need to know and experience that they are important and are seen as unique individuals. Consequently, staff should be aware of the control and power that they exercise over the life of the resident or day centre member.

Frequently, it is the attitude and low expectations of staff towards the individual with dementia that create difficulties. Expecting the person not to be able to wash, dress, or feed themselves leads to a response where the member of staff does these things for the person. It is true that some individuals with dementia will require physical assistance. However, taking time to find out what the person is still capable of and wants to do can alleviate many behaviour difficulties. Think how frustrating it is for each of us when another person takes over a task that we are capable of doing without checking if we can do it. It may make the person doing it feel they are doing a good job, but does little for our self-esteem or feeling of being in control. The experience is no different for many people with dementia. Difficult behaviour in care settings is often the person's response to how they are responded to by staff.

Communicating

At the core of all our relationships with others is the ability to communicate effectively. How staff communicate with the person with dementia is the key to unlocking understanding. Whilst dementia affects the ability of the person to participate in conversation, as this demands concentration, memory and reasoning, communication is more than words. It is the ability to engage in a meaningful way with another, which demands trust, security, and being at ease. It may involve personal contact: at times, a glance, the touch of a hand or a smile create a more powerful connection than any amount of words.

Eighty per cent of our communication is non-verbal – by eye contact, facial expression, body posture and gesture. We take cues and make judgements about being listened to and whether we should continue our conversation based on these. Should the listener have a bored expression or a negative body posture, such as turning away and looking in another direction, we will get the message that the person is not interested. Nothing has been spoken but this information influences how we feel and act in the relationship. The same can be true for people with dementia.

It is through communicating that care workers can begin to anticipate potential areas of conflict for the resident in the routine of the care home. In many homes, conflicts arise around mealtimes, intimate care tasks, and going to bed and rising.

Understanding and being understood

There is often meaning behind everything that a person with dementia says or does. Words and sentences that convey ideas that seem to make no sense may be important in telling us something about what that person is feeling and thinking. The words may be jumbled up or used incorrectly, and may refer to memories from years past as if they happened yesterday. Staff should endeavour to interpret and understand what is being communicated. This can be helped by knowledge of the person's previous culture and lifestyle, and also by recognising some of the key words that they might use to express a particular feeling. As an interpreter, the staff member should assume responsibility for clarifying what is meant and try to aid understanding by using visual prompts.

When things are still not clear, rather than cause further frustration and distress for the person, just apologise and, later, share ideas with colleagues about what may have been meant. Do not make assumptions that because a previous response worked in a previous situation that it will work every time.

Speech and language

Recognising the differences between speech and language, and expressive and receptive language can aid communication. Speech is the ability to articulate words whilst language is the ability to assemble words in a particular order that express a thought or idea. Dementia impairs both of these functions. Words and their meanings are forgotten, and communication is affected by the person's inability to reason or express themselves properly. Concentration also diminishes, making it difficult for the person to unravel long sentences, keep a track of conversations or just remember what it is they are trying to say. Where spoken English is not the language of birth but a second learned language, dementia can cause the person to return to using their first learned language, giving staff additional communication problems.

A person with dementia who has an ability to articulate clearly often deceives staff into thinking that there is no communication problem. The person may be saying the words well but the words used do not accurately express their thoughts or feelings.

EXPRESSIVE LANGUAGE

Expressive language refers to the ability to be understood. Some people with dementia develop aphasia. This is when they lose the ability to find the right word to express a thought or idea, or have difficulty putting a sentence in the correct grammatical order. The person may misuse words, substituting words of similar meanings or sounds for the intended words, such as 'son' for 'husband' or 'mouse' for 'house'. Elaborate phrases may be used for a single word in an effort to express a single thought. The 'brown carry thing' might mean handbag or case. The person may revert to using jargon words from their former occupation. To express a feeling of wanting to be left alone, one gentleman would say to staff, 'Please go to the next wicket. This station is closed'. He had been a bank teller for forty years and had also played cricket. The care worker knew that he wanted to be left alone. For some individuals, language may become so impaired that what they say is a repetition of a particular phrase such as, 'That's it, Jean!' or become a sentence or jumble of near-words that is called a 'word salad'.

Staff have to rely on their understanding of the context in which the person is trying to express themself. Particular attention should be paid to the tone of voice or facial expression, and staff need to develop a skill in narrowing the subject down through well-informed guesses.

Some practical ways to aid understanding are:

- Learn the vocabulary that the person uses.
- Recognise the difference between learned phrases, based on social pleasantries, poetry and songs, and communication that demands reasoning and word-finding ability.
- Focus on the feeling behind the words. For some people, the choice of words is not within their control, so swear words and strong emotive language may actually be expressing pleasure and enjoyment, or anger.

RECEPTIVE LANGUAGE

Receptive language refers to the ability to understand language and make an appropriate response. Many people with dementia will retain an understanding until late into the illness, even though their ability to express themselves verbally may be impaired. Determining how much understanding the person has can become apparent by noting whether they point to a specific object when given a choice, their ability to follow simple instructions such as 'please stand up' or 'pick up your spoon', or if they respond to simple 'yes' or 'no' questions.

Dementia may cause impediments to understanding because:

- The context is not clear. Misunderstandings can arise because the person fails to grasp the thread of conversation, which can cause a rise in tension and/or irritability.
- The meaning of certain words that are spoken are no longer recognised. Staff may have to rely more on non-verbal cues such as gestures, flash cards, drawings or the actual object being presented.
- Distractions interfere with the person's ability to listen. Many sitting rooms are noisy places, with lots of staff movement and the radio or television on in the corner. This can affect understanding.
- Short-term memory loss leads to only bits of information being retained, usually what has been said last.

Some practical tips

Staff should always approach the person with dementia in an open, friendly and gentle manner, even if the situation demands urgency or has caused an upset. If staff are tense and anxious, the person will probably respond by becoming tense and anxious. Staff should:

- cue the person by saying their name or who they are;
- ensure that they have the person's attention;
- give full attention to the spoken words but focus on the feelings behind the words;
- try and limit distractions;
- speak slowly (not childlike) and not patronise or speak down to the person;
- use physical gestures to enhance verbal communication;
- avoid confrontation if perceived as a threat.

Mealtimes

For people in care homes or attending day care, mealtimes are an important focal point in the day's routine and are generally social occasions. Past memories of sharing meals with family or other people will be remembered, although, for some, mealtimes may have been a solitary experience.

> **Mr Evans** comes to the dining room, but staff know that unless the food is on his plate at the table, he will not sit down. Usually, after a few minutes, he will get up, walk out of the room and refuse to come back.

What time a person had their main meal of the day, where the meal was eaten and what was eaten is subject to personal preference, which should be catered for. The timing of meals and the menu should be more about the person's needs and preferences than those of the cook or chef. It is crucial to get to know people's individual likes and dislikes: knowing, for example, that Mr Evans does not like cabbage and making sure that it is not on his plate avoids staff facing an angry Mr Evans. Having food he likes may also encourage him to stay in the dining room.

Too much noise or busyness can add to disorientation and anxiety, and be another reason for residents not remaining in the dining room. The emphasis should be on creating a relaxed, sociable setting. If at all possible, staff should sit with residents or day care clients and encourage conversation during the meal so it becomes a shared experience rather than a routine to be completed quickly. Some residents may need prompting and this should be done with a minimum of fuss. Other residents will follow the example of a staff member but sensitivity to maintaining the independence and dignity of all residents should lead to prompting only when necessary rather than taking over and feeding the person.

Some residents may require:

- A single table slightly apart from the group if their behaviour is upsetting to other residents. This is not a form of banishment from the group: it preserves some dignity for the individual and makes the mealtime less stressful. However, it may be important for someone to sit with the person if they prefer company.
- Finger food and 'snacking' because of personal preference or being unable to sit for any length of time at a meal. Finger food can be likened to a buffet-style meal.
- A careful watch to be kept on their nutritional intake and weight, particularly if they walk about a lot or eat finger food. High protein drinks may be necessary.
- Cutlery with thicker handles to help with grip, and plates with clip-on plateguards to stop food dropping off. For residents with poor co-ordination, or stiff and painful joints, these aids can help them remain independent and continue to carry out an activity of daily living. An occupational therapist can give advice and guidance.
- Help to choose what they would like to eat by being shown the food or allowed to have a taste.
- Time to go at their own pace.

Intimate care

The routine of a care home, and to a lesser extent of a day centre, may frequently mean that those caring tasks, such as being taken to the toilet, dressed/undressed and bathed, are regarded as necessary chores. It can be difficult for the care worker to think what it must be like for people when these intimate care tasks are carried out.

Personal hygiene is one area where there is unlimited scope for embarrassment and distress. Intimate care involves activities that cross the boundaries of acceptable behaviour outside the residential care setting. People do not normally expect to be escorted to the toilet, or supervised whilst naked in a bath, or undressed by a 'stranger' (member of staff).

Sensitive forward planning and being flexible will help to reduce anxiety and disorientation. Planning bath times means:

- Residents choose a bath time that fits in with their previous routine. They also choose whether help is required and whether it is a male or female member of staff who assists.
- Privacy and dignity should be respected by closing bathroom doors and not forgetting about the resident left in the bathroom.
- Ensuring that the bathroom is warm enough and the right towels and soap are provided.
- Providing an opportunity for the residents to do as much for themselves as they wish.
- Hoists and other bath aids are in working order and that the resident is not unduly anxious about using these.
- Allocating time to ensure that the bath time is relaxing and as stress-free as possible.
- Checking that the resident understands what is to happen and that they are listened to – especially if they prefer a shower.

Help with going to the toilet

It is assumed that all people with dementia are incontinent because of the illness. Although loss of bladder and bowel control does affect some people, particularly later in the illness, dementia is not always the direct cause of incontinence. Frequently, the problem the person experiences is not knowing where the toilet is located and/or remembering what to do when they reach it. Toileting programmes are a planned way of ensuring that the person is prompted to go. Some people will require physical support to get to the toilet, so it is crucial that support is offered early enough.

Eating problems

Some people with dementia may lose the swallowing reflex because of the illness. That may not be the reason, however, for a person refusing to eat or swallow: they may be having other difficulties, which will influence how they feel about eating, such as being ill or in pain, or having dentures that have not been cleaned or fitted properly. Guidance from a speech therapist will help identify the reasons for the difficulties and offer ways of helping the person.

Going to bed and rising

Getting ready for bed and deciding when to get up in the morning is a personal preference for all of us. We all have set times and routines and rituals that we follow before we go to bed. We all get up at different times in the morning, depending on what we have to do that day. There is no right or wrong. Residents with dementia are no different. Some residents will have worked shifts in their earlier years so may resent going to bed early. Others will welcome the chance to get to bed early.

Too much stimulation prior to going to bed can have an adverse effect on helping someone sleep. Consideration by staff as to how they might create the right atmosphere to help the person wind down is important. This can be done in various ways:

- In the lounge or sitting area used before bedtime, mark that the day is changing and coming to an end, by switching on table lamps and closing the curtains.
- Supper should be provided and staff can talk with residents about the day that has passed. Soothing music can help residents relax.

- Encourage residents to carry out their own nightly routine, such as having a milky drink or reading a book.

The emphasis should be on helping each person do what works best for them. This is not always easy when there are other residents to consider but not all will require assistance. Some residents often get up during the night and it is important to recognise that, for them, going back to bed may be like doing it for the first time.

KEY POINTS

- The behaviour of the individual is frequently a response to how staff respond in a particular situation.
- Understanding the person increasingly depends on care workers becoming interpreters of actions and communication.
- Routines should be flexible enough to accommodate people's likes and dislikes.
- Intimate caring tasks should be done in a way that preserves dignity and respect for the individual.

EXERCISE

Two care staff knocked on Mr Jamieson's bedroom door, entered, announced in loud voices that it was bath time, pulled the bedclothes off his bed, and began to get his soap and towel ready. Mr Jamieson responded by shouting out that he was being attacked. He physically lashed out at one of the staff and refused to leave his room.

What reasons might explain why Mr Jamieson behaved like this?

7 Dilemmas and challenges

Objectives:

- *To consider responses to particular challenges and risks that arise in group/day care*

- *To understand the needs of people with dementia, including sexual, spiritual, ethnic and cultural needs, the needs of younger people with dementia, and the needs of residents in the later stages of the illness*

- *To briefly outline legal aspects*

Maintaining ordinary life experiences for people with dementia presents staff with dilemmas and challenges. The major challenge is to see the person in the context of their whole life experience.

> **Miss Brown** has lived in the care home for five years, yet every morning she awakens very angry. She shouts at her care worker, 'This is not my home! Take me home now! Get my suitcase and coat – I need to go home now!' Yvonne, her new care worker, suggested that they go for breakfast and a cup of tea, to which Miss Brown shouted, 'My dear – you have not listened to a word I have said – I want to go home!'

Miss Brown, despite her dementia, is acutely aware that the building she lives in is not her memory of her home. These 'windows of lucidity' present a major dilemma for Yvonne, as her response needed to take account of Miss Brown's feelings. To assume that because some-one has dementia any answer will do, can make things worse, as Yvonne discovered.

Many residents express feelings or behave in a particular way as a response to being ignored, patronised or treated in a childlike manner. Present behaviour is frequently an expression of past routines and habits, which challenges our understanding. Staff need to see the person in the context of their work status, relationships, personal biography and interests. The development of a life story work or reminiscence work (see Chapter 2) can be crucial in gaining this understanding of particular habits and routines.

Group care and the individual

Achieving a meaningful routine for any one individual, whilst taking account of others, is important. Helping staff, relatives and other professionals understand the reasons for particular working practices of the home or day centre can go some way to establishing a consistent caring experience for those with dementia. People do not choose those with whom they share and it is unrealistic to expect each person to always get on well with the other people. It should not be a surprise when conflicts of interest arise, such as over what is acceptable risk or acceptable behaviour, for example. Conflicts also frequently occur when people express strong feelings or attitudes, particularly with regard to sexuality, spirituality or ethnicity.

Making the right response demands a sensitivity and awareness on the part of staff. Providing exactly what one person needs, without taking away from someone else, involves compromise, whether with one person or a group of people.

Making decisions

Many people with dementia have a strong sense of independence and can express their likes and dislikes of particular foods, colours, clothes and people. Some will still express personal opinions about a whole range of matters. Other residents will become more cautious than before because they fear making mistakes. They may even withdraw from giving any opinion, leading staff to think that they are unable to make a decision.

All residents have a need to maintain a continuity of doing familiar things, using familiar problem-solving strategies and engaging in social behaviours and activities from their past. However, it is when the resident makes decisions that pose risks for themselves that creates the major difficulties for staff. These are risks not only associated with behaviour but also how the person spends their money or recognises their need for medical help.

It is important to acknowledge that dementia does cause impairment of insight and understanding. Insight is the awareness that we all have about every aspect of our life. We know when we feel ill and can usually decide how serious it is and seek medical help. Similarly, we know when a particular action might cause us to be at risk. Understanding is based on how we perceive things, grasp their significance and remember. For many people with dementia, they may initially seem to understand but forget the consequences of their actions.

Miss Martin is due her annual flu injection but, when the nurse arrives, she becomes very angry and tells the nurse very firmly, 'I do not want the jab – I am not ill'.

The nurse faces a dilemma in determining whether the decision exercised by Miss Martin was the right one. A flu injection may be desirable but the nurse does not have the right to force Miss Martin to accept the treatment. The situation would not necessarily be different with a serious illness. It might be tempting to rush into demanding treatment in every case and seeking the legal powers to do so.

To balance the duty to care (that is, not to neglect the resident) and the duty not to make the person undergo distressing or painful treatments without good reason is very difficult. Legally, the balance has been towards the duty to care. In general, staff are protected if they take action in good faith to help residents to avoid distress, suffering or injury, even if this means actions which, in other circumstances, would be seen as interference.

Every situation is different and it is unwise to have a blanket approach. It is the effect on the individual resident and their family that is the main consideration. There is no legal power to force residents to accept treatment. Later in this section, we will consider the separate laws that exist to deal with both financial matters and care and treatment.

Risk

Many staff feel that the care home should offer 24-hour risk-free care. Sometimes this is a response to the unrealistic expectations of relatives, who think that the person will be constantly under staff surveillance, be safe and at no risk, and be better cared for than if they were at home. These unrealistic expectations can arise when relatives feel sadness and guilt about the person being in a care home. It is important to give time to relatives to share these feelings but not allow their expectations to limit the opportunities for residents.

Residents in any group care setting can get themselves into situations that pose a risk. Risk is not only associated with personal actions but other residents' behaviour and the layout of the building. Group care is usually in an unfamiliar building, designed in a way that is not like home. The resident may seek to recreate experiences from their past, which places them at risk. Each situation that arises will pose staff the challenge of whether to accept the risk, provide support to lessen the risk or to take control of the situation.

Some of the demands (although not necessarily the solutions) for a risk-free environment are:

1 Locked doors, so that the resident cannot leave the home, as this will keep them safe.

2 Restricting the involvement of the resident in the practical tasks of dressing, feeding, and daily chores.

3 Using tagging, video cameras and passive alarms so that staff know where a resident is or what they are doing.

These risks are about the balance between the duty to protect and the liberty of the person with dementia as an adult with the same rights as anyone else. The danger is that, what is seen by some as a solution, actually creates another problem:

1 Locking a door for the person with dementia means they cannot open it, yet they see others come and go. The person may get anxious or angry, or stand shaking the door all day long. There may also be safety issues concerned with fire regulations and locked doors.

2 Restricting involvement can lead to increased frustration or dependence, with the person refusing to co-operate.

3 These surveillance devices can create knee-jerk reactions, with all staff running to the sound of a buzzer or alarm. This can increase the anxiety of all residents.

However, it is unrealistic to expect a resident to adopt a lifestyle where they sit around all day, every day and show no interest in going outside. There is no substitute for staff knowing the residents' habits and preferences, and for good caring practice.

No staff member should make a decision on their own to restrain any resident in any way when thinking they are at risk. Alternatives should be considered first. If restraint is to be considered, staff need to take account of the views of the resident, the family and other professionals. Any dissenting views need to be carefully noted, as well as a record of what action has been agreed. If restraint is used, it should be the minimum necessary. Such decisions have to draw the fine line between kindly restraint, which is not cruel, and giving careful consideration to alternatives that allow residents to decide for themselves, as far as possible.

Expression of sexuality

Just because someone has dementia, it does not mean that they will not have sexual feelings. Many residents still continue to be interested in sex, want to be sexually active, and have sexual needs.

Expression of sexuality is a demonstration of need. Sexuality is not just about sexual intercourse but also about relationships, close contact, kissing, hugging and talking. People with dementia still have needs for this but they may simply mistake the appropriate time, place or person. People, who would never have dreamt of doing so in the past, may now approach strangers as they would a sexual partner. Cultural differences will also lead to certain behaviour being acceptable or regarded as taboo.

Some behaviour of residents in care homes can cause other residents, relatives and staff to be alarmed, embarrassed and disgusted, for example:

- getting into bed with other residents;
- masturbating in public;
- stripping off all their clothes in the sitting room;
- seeing a care worker as their wife/husband;
- misinterpreting intimate caring tasks such as bathing or toileting;
- gently rubbing their hand up and down the care worker's leg when being assisted in or out of bed.

Recognising that previous behaviour can still influence the resident now is crucial in developing an understanding. Some women may have been subject to sexual abuse when younger or in their marriage and this may now create difficulties.

In all situations where there is sexual activity, the following three questions should be considered:

1 What made the resident behave in this way?
2 Why was the behaviour regarded as a problem?
3 What were the consequences of the behaviour?

As well as asking the right questions, there is the further problem of some staff member's reluctance to talk about sex, often because they are uncomfortable in using certain words to discuss matters. It is important to create an environment in which staff can routinely talk about these matters. Staff also need to talk about and confront their own feelings and taboos concerning sexuality, including homosexuality, as these attitudes will influence their caring responses. It is crucial that the manager takes the lead in making this a topic of easy discussion, so that staff learn how to talk about it. Decide which words are appropriate; generally the more straightforward terminology is best.

A firm lead may be needed to prevent embarrassed giggles or the inappropriate use of language.

Spiritual needs

Spiritual awareness and needs can help all of us understand and find a meaning for life, and give us a sense of hope and personal identity. For some people, there is a strong religious component to this aspect of life. Others will strive to satisfy these needs by alternative means and challenge established practice. A useful way of helping care staff meet a person's spiritual needs is to think about aspects of the routine that combine celebration, commemoration and compassion:

- Celebration involves more than active enjoyment and feelings of pleasure. It can be to visit someone and give flowers which, both by sight and by smell, remind them of a pleasant memory of their past happiness and lead to their present enjoyment. Celebrating appropriate religious festivals, such as Christmas, Ramadan or the Feast of Atonement, can help individuals retain a sense of their cultural identity.

- Commemoration involves ritual, and the repeating of familiar songs, well-loved stories, poetry and hymns. The use of artefacts, such as a rosary or crucifix for Roman Catholics, a bible or hymn book for Protestants, and a prayer mat for Muslims, also help. Opportunities for quiet reflection or prayer are often forgotten, yet these familiar, long-standing traditions may be very important to the person with dementia, who is unable to express what they are missing. It can help to know whether the person:
  - regularly attended a place of worship;
  - prayed at certain times of the day;
  - prayed alone or with others, and if a shrine was required.

- Compassion involves a readiness to enter into the world of the person with dementia to try and show an understanding and genuine care. People often have strong views and preferences regarding religion, and these are not always predictable. Spiritual and religious nurture increases hope and the sense that all is well and will be well.

Residents who receive spiritual nurturing do appear, for a time, to have a sense of peace and be less restless. In helping to meet spiritual needs, the care worker is sustaining deeper memory.

Ethnic minority groups

A person's cultural background can affect their response and experience of being in a group care setting. Issues such as privacy and involvement in group activity and the relationships people make may be directly influenced by their customs and traditions. Some people may have been living in a close-knit ethnic community, where it was not necessary to learn English or mix with other nationalities. Others may have tried to adopt a British way of life and gained employment but have been subjected to racial abuse and intolerance. For care homes that provide support to people with dementia from different cultures, it can help, wherever possible, to recruit staff from the same ethnic groups so that there is an understanding of the culture.

Relationships with other residents and staff can accentuate cultural differences. Communication may not be in English, as people revert to the language of their home country. Residents from the Caribbean or Asia may expect staff to give them the respect that traditionally comes with age in their culture. Others may insist on adhering to strict dress codes. Muslim women may not associate with men in the public areas. Consequently, a common sitting room for both men and women may become an area where residents become stressed. Intimate caring tasks, such as being undressed and taken for a bath, might also add to difficulties for staff. People from some Middle Eastern and Asian countries may only take a shower and may not want to get in to a bath.

The increasing cultural diversity in some homes means that residents not from the UK are likely to express needs that require a knowledge and appreciation of their culture. Dementia does not rob people of their life experiences and they may become extremely upset if, for example, they see food being prepared or served in an unfamiliar way. Similarly, in some cultures, certain food may only be eaten at particular festivals during the year. To smell and taste food associated with that festival at the wrong time of year may cause further disorientation and provoke an angry response. Maintaining relationships with family members, who can help the resident keep up particular customs or prepare special food, assumes a greater importance.

Younger people with dementia

Younger people with a diagnosis of dementia can be the 45-year-old businessman, or the 27-year-old mother with AIDS, or the 51-year-old person with Down's Syndrome. Because there may not be age-appropriate care home provision for younger people, they can be placed for respite care with older people with dementia. This can lead to particular dilemmas and demands being made of staff.

> **Mr Thomson** is a 49-year-old ex-accountant with Alzheimer's disease, who has been placed in the local care home to give his wife and family a break. In the lounge of the home with older people, he insists on trying to help the older residents. He objects to staff assisting him with dressing and continually demands that he be allowed to do his work. He wants to know why he is with people who have grey hair and says he is too young to die.

Mr Thomson may have the same needs as other people with dementia but has significant differences associated with his lifestyle and age. When dementia appears in younger people, future hopes and life plans are dashed, yet he is seeing the images of ageing every day in front of his eyes. For him, it would be crucial for staff to:

- work to assist him retain his mobility, skills and strength;
- identify different coping strategies to find solutions for his problems;
- maintain his family relationships, wider social contacts and networks;
- sensitively help him in retaining a positive self-image;
- explain the meaning of his condition.

Age-appropriate activity becomes crucial, and making use of community facilities such as swimming pools and gymnasiums, pubs and clubs are ways of doing this. Linking a befriender of the same age can help maintain contact with the wider community. This approach can also take account of any diversity in culture and language.

Legal matters

Some people with dementia, who have impaired insight, difficulty in understanding and in communicating decisions, become the subject of legal interventions concerning financial matters and/or their care and welfare. These different laws provide for decisions to be made by someone else on behalf of a person with regard to their financial and property matters, or their care and treatment, including medical treatment. Financial matters include decisions about who should collect their pension, pay for their accommodation, deal with property or handle large investments. Examples of decisions about physical and medical care are where someone should live, who they have contact with or whether to have medical treatment.

However, over the past few years, the government in the UK has been reviewing the laws concerning people who lack the capacity to make decisions (the rights and protection for adults with incapacity). An objective of any new legislation is likely to stress the importance for people with dementia of being given the opportunity to express their current wishes and feelings on particular matters. This may require the assistance of an independent interpreter or an advocate, for example, and possible input about the person's previous feelings from someone who knew them well.

As any new legislation will be implemented at different times throughout the UK, and may take different forms, it is advisable to check the current situation locally before embarking on any of these procedures. A Mental Health Officer (Approved Social Worker) from the local authority or their legal department may be able to give up-to-date advice.

Decisions about financial matters

Making a will

The resident must have the required mental capacity (sometimes called 'being competent') in order to make a will. The test of capacity, in order to execute a legally binding will, is that the person (known as the testator or testatrix) must have an understanding of the effect of the will, the extent of their assets and an understanding of any claims that might be made against their estate, by a spouse or dependent, for example. It is also important that the person is not placed under undue pressure, either about the making of the will or its contents. Where a question arises about whether someone is able to make a will, a medical opinion may be necessary to make sure they are competent. Staff must not allow themselves to be named as beneficiaries and should consult their manager if this is suggested. It is probably advisable for the person to be referred to a solicitor to draw up the will, especially if their assets are complicated or if there is a question about whether the resident has sufficient capacity.

Collection of social security benefits

- Agency
  This method is for people who still have mental capacity and who want someone else to collect their social security benefits for them, perhaps because they are unable to get out themselves.

  Under social security law, the person can nominate someone – called an agent – to collect their benefits for them, but not to spend it. The nomination is an informal arrangement between the individual and the agent. The arrangement is no longer valid if the person loses mental capacity.

- Appointeeship
  Most local authority's Registration and Quality Assurance Teams require arrangements to be in place to manage the money of residents with dementia. Appointeeship is an arrangement under social security regulations, where the benefits agency appoints someone else to exercise the resident's rights to make claims for, and to

receive, social security benefits, and to spend them on behalf of the resident. The effect is that the appointee stands 'in the shoes of' the claimant; they can receive money, bring an appeal etc. They will be responsible for making sure that all benefits are claimed and the right information is given, and they have a duty to the claimant to use the money only for their benefit.

This method should be used only if the person is mentally incapacitated. It should never be used solely because the person is physically incapacitated, or for reasons of convenience.

Guidance to Benefits Agency staff emphasises that managers of homes should only be appointed as a last resort, if no suitable person (such as a relative and friend) can be found. If the manager is appointed, the Benefits Agency should inform the Registration Unit that inspects the home. The manager should keep a record of the transactions made on the resident's behalf and account for them separately.

Powers of Attorney and Enduring Powers of Attorney

Both a Power of Attorney and Enduring Power of Attorney allow a resident, by signing a legal document in prescribed form, to give someone the power to act on their behalf in financial affairs (this includes property, shares, money transactions etc). It can be either to deal with financial matters generally or limited to a specific financial transaction, such as selling a house. In order to sign, the resident must have the mental capacity to grant a power of attorney: they should understand what they are doing, what their affairs consist of and who is being given authority to act as their attorney. Managers, relatives and solicitors may need to consult a doctor about the person's mental capacity before proposing that they sign such a document.

There are two types of power of attorney that can be granted. An ordinary Power of Attorney is only valid whilst the person who made it has mental capacity. It is not valid if the person becomes mentally incapacitated and should not be used in that situation.

An unlimited Enduring Power of Attorney is also valid whilst the person who made it has mental capacity and, in addition, will continue with full effect, even if the person no longer has mental capacity, provided it has been registered with the Public Guardianship Office. The position in Scotland is different where, under the Adults with Incapacity (Scotland) Act 2000 (referred to as the '2000 Act'), new provisions for a continuing power of attorney came into force in April 2001.

Orders of the Court

England and Wales, Scotland and Northern Ireland have different legal structures and systems in place to enable someone to be appointed by the court to manage the financial affairs (including property) of someone with dementia, who does not have mental capacity. Usually this is done when a resident can neither manage their affairs nor instruct someone else or is being exploited. In England and Wales, the person appointed is called a receiver. Depending on the value of the estate (money, shares, property etc), it may not be necessary for a receiver to be appointed. Instead, the Court of Protection may issue a Direction or a Short Order authorising the person's assets to be used in a certain way for their benefit. Note that the arrangements are different in Scotland and Northern Ireland. In addition, further Parts of the '2000 Act' will come into force in Scotland from April 2002.

It is advisable that anyone who wishes to handle another person's assets should have the appropriate legal authority to do so, for example by being an attorney or receiver. Where it seems that someone is not acting in the best interests of the person with dementia (who does not have mental capacity), it may be appropriate to speak to a solicitor, who can then consider what would be the most appropriate course of action to protect the person's interests, if necessary by making an application to the court.

Decisions about care and treatment

Many people with dementia agree with (or, more often, can not or do not actively object to) decisions about their care and treatment. Decisions are often made by others on the basis that it is in the 'best interests' of the person. There is always danger of coercion, however, particularly when there are serious concerns about the person being at risk. Where any proposed course of action is clearly contrary to the wishes of the person, it may be appropriate to consider whether that person should have the opportunity to be separately advised about their position.

In Scotland, a new welfare power of attorney has been introduced under the '2000 Act', which will allow a person to be appointed to take decisions about a person's personal welfare.

Guardianship

Guardianship is a compulsory order made by the court under the Mental Health Act (Mental Health Act England and Wales 1983, Mental Health Act Scotland 1984, Mental Health Order Northern Ireland 1986). The order requires two doctors to agree that a resident is suffering from a mental disorder, and it must also be necessary to make the order in the interests of the person's welfare or for the protection of others. The order can decide where someone lives, can require them to attend somewhere, such as a day centre or clinic, and can require them to allow access to named people. It does not cover consent to treatment. For this, other sections of Mental Health legislation would need to be used; details are available from the local Mental Health Officer. The guardian can be any individual considered suitable by the court but it is usually a social worker.

Living Wills or Advance Directives

An advance directive is a record made by someone who has mental capacity about what they want to happen about their medical treatment in the event that, at some point in the future, they lose the mental capacity to decide for themselves. In addition, a living will often expresses a wish that another person be involved in decisions about the individual's treatment and/or names someone to be contacted in an emergency. You may occasionally come across a resident who has made one of these arrangements. Although there is currently no statutory authority for advance directives, following a number of court decisions and authoritative government statements, they have been recognised as having legal authority, provided that they are clear and applicable to the circumstances. In other situations, when a person is not able to make a decision on a health issue, such as having an operation, the law has established that a decision must be made by the medical practitioner in the best interests of the individual. An indication as to the resident's view may help the doctor to make the decision, and relatives, friends or carers may be able to assist as to what would be the resident's wishes in this respect.

Do not assume that people with dementia are less likely to want treatment than anyone else. Many younger people, imagining the deterioration, distress and burden of dementia, think that they would want to be allowed to die. The reality is that, although dementia is distressing for relatives and other carers, it is not always distressing for the person.

Complaints procedure

The National Health Service and Community Care Act 1990 requires each local authority to have a complaints procedure. Consequently, the authority's Registration and Quality Assurance Team will expect all care homes to have procedures, which record all complaints that residents may have concerning any aspect of their care. A written log should be kept, stating what was done about a particular complaint and whether this was resolved to the resident's satisfaction. Where the matter remains unresolved, the care home should report the complaint to the local Inspection Team. In appropriate cases, they may also wish to ensure that the individual has access to independent advice and support about their situation, for example by putting them in contact with an advocacy scheme.

Feedback from residents and relatives about the care provided should be seen as an ongoing process by staff and part of a culture of open communication, despite being more difficult for people with dementia.

Supporting people in the later stages of dementia

For people in the later stages of the illness, behaviour such as anxiety, restlessness, aggression, or shouting and screaming can be an indication that basic needs are not being addressed. Physical needs and feelings such as hunger, thirst, being too hot or too cold, feeling unsafe, uncomfortable or insecure in the environment, must be satisfied to avoid distress to the person which might result in behaviour that appears 'difficult'. Particular attention should be given to medical matters.

Residents in the later stages of the illness may become physically inactive. Although the person may be awake and their eyes open, they are not focused on a particular event or person. There may be occasional short periods of dozing or napping but they are easily roused. This apparent withdrawal may be a result of the illness but care workers should always try to have activities that engage the person for however limited the time or concentration span. Activities may need to be more of a one-to-one stimulation as opposed to group activity. A range of different activities may have to be used, including some with less reliance on spoken word:

- informal, social opportunities over a cup of tea;
- spending time in meaningful interaction with the person;
- simple physical exercise;
- listening to music;
- sensory objects to touch, look at or smell;
- massage;
- rummaging box/bag.

A regularly updated care plan can help identify how these needs will be met and, importantly, give cues to staff of the support required.

KEY POINTS

- People with dementia should be supported in their decision making.
- Staff have to find the balance between the duty to protect and the liberty of the person with dementia.
- Restraint is a last resort approach.
- Account has to be taken of cultural influences and attitudes to spirituality and sexuality.
- Younger people have a need for age-appropriate responses.
- Legal requirements should be balanced with the need for individualised care approaches.
- In the later stages of the illness, residents should have activities that offer a range of experiences.

EXERCISE

Mrs Audrey Smythe spent 10 years with her husband in India in the British Embassy. She loves opera, is a keen gardener, speaks three languages and has impeccable manners. She refuses to participate in activities such as sing-alongs, exercise times and dominoes. She also refuses her evening meal at 5pm and then complains of being hungry. She is having difficulties with her continence but gets angry when care workers remind her to go to the toilet.

What aspects of Mrs Smythe's social background might make her not feel at home in a care home?

Knowing what little you do about Mrs Smythe, what would you attempt to incorporate into her care plan?

8 Feelings of loss, pain and palliative care

Objectives:

- *To encourage a recognition that people with dementia can experience feelings of loss, grief and pain*

- *To encourage a holistic approach to the person when in the later stages of the illness*

Experiencing feelings of loss and grief

Many people have conflicting and confusing emotions when they experience major, sometimes even minor, changes in their lives. For people with dementia, who are brought in to group care for the first time, these emotions can be more akin to feelings of loss, as they experience a detachment from their past. They may grieve for the loss of their family and close friends, the loss of their familiar routine or role, or their loss of control. Their behaviour in expressing those feelings needs to be seen as part of a grieving process and not the symptoms of dementia.

> **Mr Ho** has been in a home for two weeks. Staff continually find him going into other residents' rooms and rummaging about their possessions. When staff try to get him out of the room, he physically resists.

Mr Ho may have been searching for something familiar from his past to help him feel less anxious. He may have been looking for his wife or family member, as he may think they are hiding from him. If he believes his wife is in the room, he will be angry at being asked to leave.

Reactions to loss can lead to fluctuations between feeling angry, frustrated, withdrawn and depressed, to, at other times, being excited, co-operative and accepting of their new living arrangements. A new set of 'significant others' has entered Mr Ho's world. Whereas his wife or daughter may have been his main carer, now there are numerous staff and 'strangers'. This may present a threatening situation, especially if his memory and reasoning are failing. Staff, in their verbal and body language, should give a clear message of acceptance and understanding and not discount such feelings. Affirming the expression of feelings of loss can provide a reassurance to the person that it is right that they feel this way. When done sensitively, it does not deny the past experience of the individual but is a response to their feelings when they arise and when the person wants to communicate.

Not everything is lost and it is a mistake to disregard the lifetime of experiences that makes the person the unique individual they are. Even in the face of many of the disabling affects of dementia, most people will:

- remember things from their distant past;
- have opinions and offer advice;
- continue with long-learned patterns of behaviour;
- learn to adapt to new routines;
- enjoy pleasurable sensory stimuli;
- respond to and express emotion;
- follow a logical train of thought.

Cultural differences exist in dealing with the experience of loss, and recognising the cultural values and behaviour associated with loss may help explain particular behaviour. Southern Mediterranean cultures, for example, often deal with loss by sharing the experience, whilst British culture tends to be less demonstrative and adopts a 'keep a stiff upper lip' attitude. Differences also exist between generations in reactions to loss.

Providing support to the family

Anticipatory grief can be the response of a partner or other family members, as they see the person with dementia change before their eyes. Members of the family see the losses associated with the illness and so mourn for the person they once knew. Relatives often talk about feeling guilty that they could not do more, which can lead to unrealistic demands of care home workers. It is important for everyone that the family is able to express its feelings in privacy with a member of staff, away from the resident.

Experiencing feelings of pain

Being in pain is an individual experience: what one person considers pain may not represent pain for another. Pain affects us differently according to the sensation, the knowledge and the emotions associated with the experience.

Consequently, the experience of pain for residents will be different, and care workers require acute observational skills to note changes. Many of the older generation were brought up in a culture that encouraged them to be stoic and not complain. This can lead older people to under-state their pain, which, in turn, will lead staff to underestimate the significance of their symptoms.

A major problem for people with dementia is how they express their pain. Differences exist in the way each person uses the language associated with pain. For a resident to hold their head in their hands and moan 'cabbage' might indicate that they have a headache. Words are only part of the way in which residents communicate their experience of pain; staff should be sensitive to individual differences in behaviour and mood. Staff should also recognise that cultural differences towards pain may increase the chance of misunderstanding.

Acute pain

When a person experiences acute pain, there are changes in that person which an observer can detect. At one level, pain is often a reason for us being intolerant or cranky. It can make us restless, or cause us to change position or fidget. The same applies to older people or those with dementia.

BODY LANGUAGE

Some clues to a person being in pain are when they:

- refuse to put weight on their lower limb, as they feel pain in their hip;
- spit out food when being fed because of toothache;
- lie with their knees drawn up, as they feel abdominal pain;
- pull away when their arm is touched, as they have a pain in their shoulder;
- hit out at the care worker when being turned in bed, as they feel pain in their back.

It is hard to distinguish between body language and behaviour, as the one blends into the other. However, it is not right to make an assumption that residents with dementia feel no pain.

PHYSIOLOGICAL CHANGES

In severe acute pain, such as in a heart attack, the person may become very pale, and sweating may occur. The blood pressure may become lowered, and the person may faint or vomit. These are referred to as 'physiological changes'.

These changes are sometimes not so obvious in much older people and so they cannot be relied on to indicate acute pain. For example, in some people the only sign of a heart attack may be the sudden onset of mental confusion.

Chronic pain

Acute pain that has been going on for a long time is termed chronic pain. The body's physiological reactions become 'worn out' or blunted. This means that the usual reactions to being in pain, such as pallor or sweating, do not occur. Staff need to listen carefully to what the resident says and note any changes in their overall wellbeing.

Over time, chronic pain can lead to the resident:

- being depressed;
- withdrawing from contact with others;
- experiencing sleep disturbance;
- having impaired mobility;
- becoming dependent on medication.

Attitudes towards pain

Residents feel pain and worry about pain as much as anyone else – it is not necessarily part of growing older or having dementia. Residents in care homes have similar aches and pains to everyone else, the most prevalent being in the joints, limbs and the back. These are due most commonly to arthritis. Although staff may think of this as a mild problem, residents most commonly describe the pain they have as being a major problem.

Many residents in care homes have fears about suffering pain. They also have attitudes that hinder adequate pain management: surveys of people living in institutional care have shown various reasons why older people do not report pain to their carers. These include:

- fear of painful investigation;
- denial — 'if I ignore the pain it may go away';
- not wanting to lose control in making decisions about their own body;
- not wanting to bother other people;
- not wanting to be thought of as a complainer;
- fear of being given drugs that may be addictive.

It is good practice to record instances when an individual is in pain, as this allows staff to follow up and to discuss possible reasons at hand-over or review meetings.

STAFF AWARENESS

There is ample evidence that people with dementia, living in care homes, do not receive appropriate treatment for pain because of the lack of staff awareness. Forgetting simple measures, such as heat packs, a good range of pillows, positioning and massage, can mean that an older person is not as comfortable as they could be when pain is present from conditions such as arthritis and rheumatism. Sometimes, if staff just remain in close proximity to the resident, that person can experience a significant reduction in their perceived pain intensity, even though the staff member does not administer any treatment.

The pain suffered by residents in long-term care does not always impact as strongly on staff as some of the other experiences and behaviour they encounter. However, to the older person in pain, the reasons are likely to be unimportant compared to the fact they are in pain, and staff should be alert to the possibilities and take appropriate action.

Palliative care for residents in the later stages of dementia

Priorities for palliative care are:

- affirming life;
- never hastening or postponing death;
- providing relief from pain and other distressing symptoms;
- preventing injury;
- offering support that responds to psychological and spiritual needs;
- offering support to any family members.

Palliative care for residents with dementia, particularly for those in the later stages, draws on the concepts of hospice care. The primary purpose of hospice care is to provide comfort and support to the patients and their families in the final stages of an illness, so they may live as fully and as comfortably as possible. Death and dying are not seen as a medical problem but a significant part of life's journey that involves the individual, their family and the community. The emphasis becomes that of maintaining a quality of life for the person.

One aspect of this quality of life in hospice care is to have adequate relief from any pain. This applies equally to residents with dementia.

However, other components of hospice care also apply to residents with dementia in care settings. Some aspects to note are:

- creating a caring community in which the emphasis is on living, caring and connecting with others;
- personalising care;
- providing symptom relief and promoting comfort;
- developing an openness and honesty with residents and families.

Residents and their family can be helped with trying to make sense of the losses they are experiencing, and the support provided should be designed to balance and satisfy basic needs, inner self needs and social needs.

KEY POINTS

- Residents experience a series of losses when admitted to a care home.
- New residents may feel threatened by unfamiliar staff and apparent 'strangers'.
- People with dementia experience pain as much as those without dementia.
- Clues to individuals being in pain can be picked up by their body language and/or changes in behaviour.
- Palliative care for people with dementia should focus on maintaining their quality of life experience.

EXERCISE

Mrs Alexis had just been to the hairdresser. The care worker was keen to help Mrs Alexis feel good about herself, so stood her in front of the mirror and commented on how nice her hair looked. Mrs Alexis became very angry, shouted at the care worker to stop playing tricks as she knew her mother was dead, and burst into tears.

Why might Mrs Alexis have behaved in this way?

9 Issues for day care

Objectives:

- *To involve the relative in devising appropriate support*
- *To provide meaningful activity that stimulates and maintains functioning*
- *To maintain a routine and rhythm to the day*
- *To consider working with groups*

Much of what has been written in earlier chapters of this book applies to people with dementia in day care, as well as those in residential care homes. Nevertheless there are certain issues in supporting people in day care that merit special attention.

Involving the carer in devising appropriate support

Many carers, particularly family carers, become physically exhausted and emotionally stressed trying to keep the person with dementia active and involved in normal life experiences. It can be extremely upsetting and discouraging for a carer when the person they once saw as capable begins to lose ability. The carer may feel frustrated that, despite all their efforts, there is no improvement. Feelings of guilt may arise because they feel unable to cope with the unremitting demands of caring. It is in such situations that attendance at a day centre or day care group is seen as offering respite.

In such circumstances, day centre staff need to be sensitive to how the carer is feeling, as much as the person with dementia. Some family carers will want information about how the dementia will progress, others may not. Some may feel that they have failed in some way at not being able to keep the person at home, even if only for a few hours. It is important for the co-ordinator to take time to explain the normal routine of day care to the person with dementia and their carer. Equally crucial is for the person with dementia to talk with their carer about what likes/dislikes and interests they have. The day care staff should try to link their support to what would benefit the ongoing caring relationship at home. This might mean:

- involving the person with dementia in activities that maintain particular skills at home;
- helping the carer develop different ways of coping with behaviour;
- devising opportunities for the carer to participate in certain activities at the day care centre, which maintains a continuity of support for the person with dementia;
- being a first point of contact to listen to any difficulties the carer might be facing.

Providing meaningful activity that stimulates and maintains functioning

Not all activities are equally appealing to every person with dementia. Identifying what activity would be meaningful for the person would be dependent on knowing something about the life experience of that individual. However, for some people with dementia, who have difficulty in understanding or expressing choice, it can help to consider the following five indicators of meaningful activity:

1 The activity should be one that the person opts to do voluntarily. No-one likes to be forced to be involved in something they do not want to do. However, staff should check first whether any initial resistance to participating is because the person has not understood what is happening, whether they are afraid of being involved, or whether it is an informed refusal.

2 There has to be a purpose to the activity, although the outcome may simply be to engage the person and/or to give them pleasure from doing it. Some activities are done because they are fun in themselves and make the person feel good. The purpose should be obvious to the person, as being asked to do something that is perceived as pointless or not enjoyable can be frustrating and demeaning.

3 The activity should be socially-appropriate, one that respects the social image that the person holds of themselves. A person who is desperately trying to hold on to a sense of competence may become distressed at being asked to do something which seems childish. Being asked to do a simple jigsaw puzzle may not offend one person but can be a grave insult to another.

4 The activity should not lead to failure. The image that the person with dementia portrays to others in a group when involved in a task can preserve their dignity. The activity should be within the capability of the person and lead to some enjoyment. Failing to correctly undertake a simple task can create much embarrassment and frustration for the individual and those around.

5 The activity should be a pleasurable experience for the person with dementia. Knowing their previous interests, hobbies and work experience can give clues as to what they might potentially enjoy but new pursuits can also be tried. Smell, taste and touch are senses that can provide pleasurable sensation. Intergenerational activities with children should not be overlooked, as these can give the person the opportunity to enjoy children's games, songs and playfulness, yet still preserve their adult demeanour.

These five indicators can help staff in determining whether a particular activity is appropriate, although, wherever possible, the choice of activity should be left to the individual. If staff encounter some resistance to participating, they should try to find out whether the person is not interested, or if they have not fully understood what is happening and need more explanation. For some people with dementia, the concept of doing something called 'activity' will be meaningless. Providing visual clues to an activity can help prompt involvement. For some activities, and to lessen any noise or confusion, it can be helpful to provide less stimulating areas: in a day care setting, it is important to try and create either a quiet corner, preferably screened off from other areas, or have a quiet room.

Maintaining a routine and rhythm to the day

For people with dementia, the familiarity of knowing what happens when they arrive at day care can alleviate anxiety or insecurity. When everything flows predictably from one activity to another, the person can begin to relax. This helps them cope with their fear of the unknown and it offers a sense of control. Routine can give confidence, aid memory and give orientation to the day. Although a person may not be able to tell the time, they instinctively know when it is lunchtime or time to go home. This rhythm to life is crucial for every individual but especially valuable for the person with dementia. The temptation to cram a lot of activities in to the programme, so that staff do not feel in a rut, should be avoided.

Working with groups

For many people with dementia, attending day care means becoming part of a group, which may not necessarily be their previous experience. For day care groups, rituals are important. Consistent and predictable cues can assist with fostering a sense of belonging to the group. The day may begin with the introductions: a particular greeting might be used or, in some instances, a welcome song that everyone sings. The song might be one that enables every group member to use their name: each time the members come together, they need to be re-introduced to each other and the staff.

Day care staff need to discuss how much control will be delegated to the people with dementia. It should be decided if the purpose of the group is for the staff to follow a range of options decided by the group members. Alternatively, if the group members will follow a range of options chosen by the staff. There is no wrong response but the aims of the day care programme need to be clearly thought out. If day care is to promote a sense of identity, by providing a social experience, and intends to establish a bond and sense of belonging to the group, then members should have opportunities to exert some control. A group that a person with dementia can thrive in is one that allows the person to just be there and participate on whatever basis they are able.

Large day care groups present particular difficulties, as the most effective group size for encouraging participation is about six or seven members. If space permits, the larger groups may be divided into smaller groups, centred on particular types of activity. Some of these activities may provide sensory stimulation, such as an aromatherapy massage, whilst others might involve more creativity, such as painting.

Particular themes can be developed that reflect the cultural diversity of members. There may, for example, be a Chinese theme week at Chinese New Year, involving dressing up in traditional costume, making hats, tasting food, and dancing. Staff can also be invited to join in. Such activities can be a stimulating experience for group members, and foster a sense of belonging.

Because dementia tends to isolate individuals, belonging to a group can lead to a positive social experience. A group can offer the opportunity to be part of something, whilst allowing individuals to maintain their unique identities. As a member of a day care group, a person can experience being with peers, find allies and friends, and gain mutual support.

However, a number of people with dementia, brought together to do a common activity, is not a group. Unless the group members somehow connect with each other, they are just people doing the same thing. This is the challenge for day care.

KEY POINTS

- Day care should support the person in maintaining daily living skills.
- Meaningful activity should be voluntary, have a purpose, be socially-appropriate, not lead to failure and be pleasurable.
- The aims and purpose of the day care programme for each person should be identified.
- Day care can provide a range of opportunities, which help the person feel less isolated and maintain their individuality.

EXERCISE

Using the 5 indicators for activity, consider how the day care activity provided at your centre provides a range of experiences for the person with dementia, and helps maintain individuality.

10 Staff teamwork

Objective:

- *To promote a teamwork approach to the support of people with dementia*

A person-centred approach and teams

If person-centred care is something that should be evident in the support of residents, it should also be evident in staff teams. Members need to value the different skills and experiences that each will bring to the team. It is equally important to recognise that providing support to residents cannot be done by one member of staff. The continuity of care is dependent on different team members maintaining a consistent approach to individual residents.

In the closed environment of a care home, the worlds of the staff and the residents interweave and inter-relate. Not only is the effectiveness of support for residents influenced by the attitudes and commitment of various team members, it is affected by the resident being co-operative in accepting certain imposed routines. Team members should be careful, however, not to exert too much power and control over the residents' lives: people with dementia can become passive recipients of well-meaning actions that, in reality, can further disable by not providing them with opportunities to use their abilities.

A role for managers

Managing teams is demanding, as it needs time and forward planning. Maintaining the skill level of individual staff members, whilst encouraging teams to develop, means recognising that each member is a mixture of feelings, attitudes, thoughts, prejudices, skills, strengths and weaknesses. This can be difficult enough to cope with but, put a group of people together, be it residents with dementia or a staff team, and the problem is even bigger.

Developing an effective team approach requires leadership and example to be shown by the manager. The manager who demonstrates and models the aspects of care with residents that they wish to see implemented will gain credibility with the team. Team members see the manager responding to situations with residents with which they have to cope. Similarly, a manager who does not always stay in their office can see the actual caring practice at the time it occurs. Adopting such a role can lead to learning opportunities and discussion concerning approaches to individual residents. Co-ordinating effort and ensuring the philosophy of care is implemented can then be based on the strengths and abilities recognised in each team member.

One aspect of the co-ordination of support is helping the team to cope with change. As the needs of residents change, so must the responses of staff. As the team develops increasing expertise, so too must the manager change how they provide support. Effective teamwork begins with the manager adopting an empowering approach towards staff.

The culture of care

Team members frequently follow routines and adopt patterns of behaviour that maintain a particular culture of care. Often it is not what is spoken about that influences care practice. Personal expectations, previous life and work experiences, as well as attitudes and beliefs about what is important for older people with dementia, combine to influence their role. The culture of care should not be dictated by the needs of the staff: residents should not have to have their evening meal by 4.30pm because the cook finishes at this time. Good dementia care means helping staff move past the 'it's just common sense' response. Sometimes conflicts arise out of a sincere desire by staff to be helpful to the person with dementia. For some, 'a need to be needed' motivates them to take responsibility away from the person with dementia, which can lead to a further loss of ability, as the person becomes more dependent.

Playing as a team

Teams do not happen by magic. Any team sport will demonstrate how each player has an assigned role that builds on their particular expertise and skill: a football manager would not ask the goalkeeper to play as a striker, for example. Managers have a crucial role in selecting and recruiting the right person for the right job. They also need to provide the right training regime and ensure that everyone performs to the best of their ability. There are obvious similarities for a care home team.

Bring a group of day centre or care home staff together and a common complaint is that of not working as a team. At times, responding to the needs of people with dementia will be stressful and daunting, especially on the occasions when things go unexpectedly wrong, despite all good caring practice and good intentions. When something goes wrong, a typical response of many teams is to:

- blame a colleague;
- feel they do not have the necessary skills;
- complain that working with people with dementia is too demanding and unrewarding, and not the caring they want to do;
- blame the management for expecting them to cope without enough staff or enough time;
- confirm their view that people with dementia are over-dependent and unpredictable.

Such views reflect the fact that care staff are often caught up in the dilemmas, pressures and responsibilities of the job. The importance of valuing each other's personal abilities as team members is forgotten. There is frequently a lack of co-ordination of effort.

The staff team of the care home or day centre is not any different to the sports team. Each member has a unique skill, a different part to play. Everyone needs to be clear about what other members are good at and what particular role they have to play. With motivation, discipline and skill, individual members can combine to achieve an effective and efficient team.

Developing team working

All too often, care workers set themselves the unrealistic objective of being all things to all people with dementia and forget that personalities can sometimes clash. It is not a positive experience for the care worker or the person with dementia if there is continual conflict.

A positive team can:

- create an atmosphere that encourages staff to develop and improve skills;
- enable staff to develop a deeper knowledge of the residents, making it easier to identify changes in behaviour;
- use their knowledge of residents to predict the resources required to meet their changing needs;
- achieve better care by working together.

Communication

Team members often communicate about the wrong things. Discussion of the day-to-day work is important but equally important is the need to stop and think about how the team is functioning.

Working with individuals with dementia can be very stressful. Staff can sometimes expend a lot of time and energy caring sensitively for the person but their efforts are met with a blank response; alternatively, staff can be taken by surprise, as the person gives vent to strong, emotional outbursts. These occasions can be tiring, and it is important for the team to talk and to give each other support. This support does not just happen – everyone in the team must have a clear sense of their purpose and agree how they will put this into practice.

Training the team

Providing training is good but, on its own, it is not a cure for the ills of poorly thought-out procedures, inappropriate routines or a lack of philosophy of care, which are the hallmarks of poor management. Unfortunately, training can often be a knee-jerk response to something having gone wrong in the home or day centre.

Managers have a vested interest in getting the training programme right. Any programme should encourage staff to learn and gain insights into their own working practice. Encouraging team members to engage in learning is more likely to be successful if it addresses their concerns and is relevant to their work setting. To make a positive impact on staff morale and working practice, a training programme needs to be ongoing over a period of time.

More important is how what is learned from the training is translated into action in the workplace, so that there is an observable difference. Such changes depend on the managers changing their practice, too. Many managers fall into the trap of expecting staff to change but do nothing to provide opportunities to help them work differently or try out new ideas. An effective training programme begins with the manager recognising a need to change how things happen, so that it becomes a team approach to learning.

Suggestions for achieving good teamwork and practical support for each other are:

- *Set up 'hand-over' meetings between shifts to evaluate and review what has happened*
Too often, hand-over meetings at the end of shifts are cursory and predictable, with little meaningful information passed on about residents. A more productive way to use the time would be to evaluate the care plan of one resident and check whether goals are being achieved or whether changes are required.

- *Arrange regular supervision on a one-to-one basis*
Supervision is essential in any programme, and for managers to work regularly with their staff on a one-to-one basis can sometimes be as important as the actual training. Encouraging staff to reflect on one

aspect of their work can promote learning. The objective is not to find fault but to use actual practice to prompt thinking about the questions: How could I have done this differently? What do I need to know more about? This, in turn, can lead to the identification of further needs and the provision of further training. A follow-up meeting within one week of any internal/external training event should be organised, so that the team member can share ideas gained from the training. This can lead to that team member facilitating a discussion with other team members.

- *Organise peer forums*

Small groups of three or four team members could arrange to meet for about 45 minutes at the end of a shift every fortnight to discuss informally some practice issues of concern. The manager need not lead this forum: team members could each take responsibility for a particular topic or, alternatively, use some group discussion material.

- *Have regular staff meetings to further team development*

Meetings should not be occasions to be endured, when only one or two people contribute and when some managers use the opportunity to lay down the rules. The quality of meetings can usually be judged by the way people either look forward to or dread the normal weekly or monthly get-together and by how much team members contribute to discussions.

- *Plan for special interest meetings*

Inviting colleagues from other fields can stimulate and improve the quality of collaborative work, as ideas and experiences are shared. Community nurses, occupational therapists and home care assistants, as well as carers of people with dementia living at home, can all add to understanding and encourage more sensitive responses.

- *Use local resources*

Local colleges and libraries can supply books and articles on subjects related to dementia. These can be reviewed and discussed by staff, so keeping in touch with current thinking and practice.

● *The developing team*

Teams often lose sight of what they are good at doing. It can be difficult for staff to know when there has been improved practice. A manager, who gives praise and comments positively on how a team has developed their working practice with residents, will help the staff feel valued. Similarly, discussion with team members concerning the care plan for a particular resident can be a time to reinforce observed good practice.

Although effective teams know what they do well, sometimes more formalised observation techniques, involving external observers, can help in identifying practice that requires development. Dementia Care Mapping (DCM) is a structured observation technique, which focuses on the experience of the resident. By observing the activity of a resident over five minutes blocks of time during a six-hour period, staff can assess if they need to make changes to their working practice. The mapping exercise will usually be repeated 3-6 months later, so that any change in practice can be noted. This is an evidence-based approach to planning the ongoing training requirements of a staff team.

● *Recognise the personal needs of staff*

Job satisfaction for many staff members comes from when the residents with dementia appreciate and gain benefit from their efforts. Providing that support and care requires a great deal of emotional energy and commitment, however, and it will not always be a happy, stress-free experience. It can be frustrating and demoralising when residents complain, are unappreciative and tell staff that they are no good at their job. Add the intensity of supporting residents, who may be constantly anxious, restless, prone to emotional outbursts and feelings of loss, and all this becomes a recipe for staff 'burn-out' and exhaustion. Managers need to be sensitive to staff needs and plan how they provide time and opportunity for them to share their feelings about their caring role.

KEY POINTS

- Team members need to value each other as much as they value residents.
- Recognise and make use of the different abilities, skills and personalities of team members to enhance overall care and support.
- Help team members cope with stress by encouraging discussion and providing training opportunities.
- Avoid having the expectation that every problem can be solved.
- Be prepared for mistakes and learn from these.

EXERCISE

Given that caring for people with dementia can be stressful, what is provided in your place of work to meet your needs?

Appendix 1

Introductory training sessions

These short training sessions are for managers to use with their staff. They are designed to help team members develop an understanding of dementia care, based on the contents of this book. Managers should enable their staff to either have their own copy or have access to a copy to read the relevant chapters before each meeting. The aim should always be to prompt staff thinking and to link the discussion back to actual working practice with people with dementia. A suggested running order, with timings for guidance, is given for the first meeting. It is important to plan meetings 2, 3 and 4 in the same detail, using the following guidelines.

Time	Meeting 1: Person-centred care and seeing the person behind the illness
	Refer to Chapters 1 and 2.
2pm	Welcome and explanation of why the meeting is called.
2.05pm	Pairs exercise. Write up the following questions on a flipchart: 1 What concerns do I have about working with people with dementia? 2 What would I want to learn more about? Ask team members to work in pairs to discuss the two questions.
2.15pm	Note all the responses on the flipchart. At this point, do not make any comment but, after each pair has responded, have the group consider if there are particular concerns that are common. Explain that you wish, as a team, to think about improving your response and understanding of people with dementia. It begins by recognising each person's unique life experience. The next exercise focuses on this.

2.30pm Individual exercise.
Recognising the importance of past life experience.

This is a visual drawing exercise, using an A4 sheet of paper. Ask each member to draw a large **S** from the top of the paper to the bottom. Explain that the **S** represents their life-line. The top of the **S** is when they were born, so mark at the tip of the **S**: 0 years. Then, along the rest of the **S**, mark off in equal sections the ages 5, 10, 15, 20, 25 etc.

On the **right side** of the line, ask each member to note down an experience they have had at different ages, starting from birth. Examples:

● 5 years old – went to school
● 12 years old – joined the Scouts/Girl Guides
● 15 years old – first Saturday job
● 21 years old – moved into a flat etc.

Allow 5 minutes.

On the **left side** of the line, ask team members to write the roles and relationships they have had from birth. Examples:

● 0 years – son/daughter
● 3 years – brother/sister
● 5 years – schoolfriend etc.

Allow 5 minutes.

2.45pm Having done this, ask each member to share their experiences with a partner and discuss the question:

● 'Do my past experiences influence me now?'

It is likely that each person will have some experience that will influence their attitude, behaviour or feeling about something.

2.55pm Share ideas.

Points to emphasise. These will likely be different for everyone but influence who we are and what relationships and life experiences are important to us. This is just as important for people with dementia.

3.05pm   Discussion exercise.
Use the questions at the end of Chapter 1. If necessary, type them out on a separate piece of paper. Give people about 5 minutes to think about the questions.

Now discuss how you might respond. Use the answer in Appendix 2 as a guide.

3.20pm   Practical exercise.
Each team member should be asked to find out what may be important for a person with dementia in their care. The objective is to try and gain clues that might help future responses and plans of action. This could be the start of life story work. Caution the team not to start something that they cannot maintain – they should respect the feelings of the person with dementia and not get themselves into a position of letting them down.

3.30pm   Agree a date for next session.

This book can provide discussion points for further meetings, as suggested below. Using the running order and timings guidance given above, you can plan meetings 2, 3 and 4 in more depth.

Meeting 2: Understanding Dementia

Refer to Chapters 3 and 4.

What is dementia and what is not dementia?
Dementia from a social disability perspective.

Meeting 3: Buildings and Behaviour

Refer to Chapters 5 and 6.

The impact of buildings.
Behaviour as a response to routines.

Meeting 4: Dilemmas and challenges

Refer to Chapters 7, 8 and 9.

Issues that arise in group care and day care:
- Feelings of loss;
- Day care issues.

Appendix 2

Learning points from discussion exercises

Chapter 1

The clues to the needs of Mr Heatherington are in the questions he asks. If he had only just moved into the home and was now separated from close family, friends and familiar surroundings, he might feel that he is being punished by being taken to a strange place. He might need reassurance that his relatives and friends will be keeping in contact: Cathy could explain where he is and when they are coming to visit. Similarly, he may have some past experience that he still remembers, and something that is happening now brings the emotion and feelings back. Knowing the previous life experience of Mr Heatherington would help Cathy to know what might be a helpful response to his questions.

It was obviously exasperating and time consuming for Cathy dealing with Mr Heatherington. Although he was making slow progress, it was important not to take over. Cathy might have helped by prompting and giving practical help only when required. She could have taken the opportunity to try and discover why he felt he was being punished. It is crucial for Cathy to establish a rapport to support the efforts of Mr Heatherington, as involving him can help foster a sense of purpose and self-esteem, and so maintain his confidence and skills. It is equally important in day care.

The routine should not take staff away from direct caring. Some staff will feel that, unless they do these chores, they are not fulfilling their role. But, if we stop and think about those who are in care homes, most will still be able to help with basic household chores. Tight time schedules for routines, such as bed making and housekeeping chores, should not assume a higher priority than contact with residents.

Chapter 2

The clue to understanding what is going on for Mrs Morales is to be clear about the importance that different cultures give to extended family relationships. For Mrs Morales, her expectation was that her son and daughter had a duty owed to her as the mother. She could not understand why they did not follow traditional responsibilities. Consequently, an approach could be to involve the family, if possible, in some of the day care activities. If not, Mrs Morales may need reassurance that her family will be keeping in touch, or visiting her at a later date.

Chapter 3

Suggested answers to the quiz:

1 Which is the most common type of dementia?
   The most common type of dementia is Alzheimer's disease. It accounts for between 40 to 45 per cent of people with dementia. Alzheimer's disease causes the degeneration of nerve cells and neurotransmitters in the brain over a period of time.

2 Is there any known cure for dementia?
   At present, there is no known cure. However, there are drug treatments for people in the earlier stages of Alzheimer's disease, which can reduce the speed of progression of the illness. Current medical research is also bringing closer the possibility of a vaccine for Alzheimer's disease.

3 Which organ of the body is most affected by dementia?
   The brain – which is the control centre of our bodies.

4 Is it easy to diagnose someone with dementia?
   No. Diagnosis is difficult because other illnesses, depression and acute confusion can mimic the symptoms of dementia.

5 Does a sudden change in behaviour mean the person has dementia?
   Not necessarily. There may be a variety of reasons, such as the person having problems with diet or a chest infection, being on new medication, being depressed or just having an 'off day'. It is important, therefore, to have a doctor give the person a thorough check-up.

6 Why are acute confusion and depression not like dementia?
Whilst many of the symptoms are similar to those of dementia, both acute confusion and depression may be treatable with medication and the person is likely to improve. Dementia is not a temporary state but a progressive illness with no cure.

7 I sometimes forget things. Do I have dementia?
Everyone has a tendency to forget sometimes. This is considered normal. For those of us who lead hectic and busy lives, we may even be more likely to misplace or forget things; we are too busy thinking about other matters. However, should you experience frequent times of memory loss for recent events, contact your doctor.

8 Is the use of medication a good idea to cope with difficult behaviour?
Medication to control behaviour should always be the last resort, after all other approaches have been tried. Many people with dementia experience more disorientation and communication difficulties when given medication.

Chapter 4

We know that Mrs Braithwaite has dementia but this does not necessarily mean that her behaviour, which is out of the ordinary, is because the dementia has got worse. The chapter suggests physical causes for deterioration in health, such as poor diet, urinary tract infection, chest infection, or strokes. It is crucial that she is checked by her GP for any physical illness. Other questions to consider are:

- Is she subject to falls at home?
- Has she been prescribed medication that she has forgotten to take, or had the dosage changed, which has caused side effects?
- Is she prone to depression?
- Is she getting enough sleep at night?

Chapter 5

£50 can do a lot. For example, toilet doors could be made more obvious by making signs with words and/or a picture of an old-fashioned toilet on the door, at the eye level of residents. To break up long corridors, curtains could be draped to the side, or wall hangings and pictures put up. A pot plant, perhaps climbing up a simple piece of garden trellis-work, can also be used to break the monotony of the corridor. Small domestic-style table lamps could be placed in sitting rooms and switched on in the evening to give a cosier glow than fluorescent lamps.

Chapter 6

It is no surprise that Mr Jamieson responded as he did. The sudden awakening, the loud voices, the grabbing hands all constitute an infringement of his personal space and dignity. His fighting back is a direct response to how he was approached. He misunderstood the actions of the care staff (whom he saw as strangers) as being an intention to harm him.

It is important for staff to respond sensitively to people with dementia, especially when carrying out intimate care tasks, such as bathing. The person should be treated with dignity and, ideally, be given the choice as to whether they would like to have a bath, when, and who they would like to assist them.

Chapter 7

An understanding of social class in the UK is as important as an understanding of religious or cultural differences. Mrs Smythe's lifestyle is likely to have been very different from that of most care workers. In providing individualised care, staff should give some thought to the behaviour associated with someone of her background. Some practical things to do would be to:

- check how she would like to be addressed;
- offer a meal later in the evening, which may have been her routine;
- explore games and activities she might enjoy: card games, scrabble, flower arranging or gardening;
- encourage her to maintain her role as a hostess, by offering her the opportunity to help with serving afternoon tea or early evening drinks.

Chapter 8

Mrs Alexis may have seen the reflection as her mother and yet realised that her mother was not there. She probably does not see herself as the grey-haired, plump woman with glasses and a wrinkled 80-year-old face: she may remember herself as a no-nonsense, efficient legal secretary, who was always in the height of fashion and certainly did not wear glasses. Although she saw the image in the mirror, she may have been reminded of the losses she had experienced in her life; or she might have been in pain. The care worker would need to spend time responding to such feelings. Having a memory or life story book as an aid can be invaluable in such circumstances.

Chapter 9

Day care should not be seen only as a means of occupying the person with social activities. Although this stimulation is important, it is also crucial to find out what people can still do for themselves and provide opportunities to help them retain such skills. The Chinese theme meal, given as an example in the chapter, only happened because some members of the group were from the Chinese community. With the support of the staff, they did the preparation, cooking and serving of the meal. This, in turn, provided a stimulating activity for others, who could watch the cooking and taste different dishes.

Chapter 10

Some well-tried ways were noted in the chapter. However, after critical incidents have occurred, make time for a de-briefing session. This can allow staff to give vent to their feelings and also provide an opportunity for them to unwind, share concerns and sort out why things happened in a particular manner. Not only can this help more consistent approaches to care to develop, it can also help identify further training needs.

Further Reading

Archibald, C. (1991 and 1992) *Activities for People with Dementia.* Dementia Services Development Centre, University of Stirling

Jackson, G. and Jacques, A. (2000) *Understanding Dementia* (third edition). Churchill Livingston, London

Zgola, J. (1999) *Care that Works: A Relationship Approach to Persons with Dementia.* John Hopkins Press, London

Garrett, S. and Hamilton-Smith, E. (1995) *Rethinking Dementia – an Australian Approach.* Ausmed Publications, Melbourne

Goldsmith, M. (1996) *Hearing the Voice of People with Dementia: Opportunities and Obstacles.* Jessica Kingsley, London

Chapman, A., Jackson, G. and McDonald, C. (1999) *What Behaviour? Whose Problem?* Dementia Services Development Centre, University of Stirling

Marshall, M. ed. (1997) *State of the Art in Dementia Care.* Centre for Policy on Ageing (CPA), London

Benson, S. and Kitwood, T. (1995) *The New Culture of Dementia Care.* Hawker Publications, London

Killick, J. and Cordonnier, C. (2000) *Openings: Dementia Poems and Photographs.* Hawker Publications, London

Powell, J. (2000) *Care to Communicate: Helping the Older Person with Dementia.* Hawker Publications, London

Useful Addresses

Action on Elder Abuse
Astral House
1268 London Road
London SW16 4ER
Tel: 020 8764 7648
Elder Abuse Response Line: 0808 808 8141 (10am-4.30pm weekdays)
Email: aea@ace.org.uk
Website: www.elderabuse.org
Aims to prevent abuse of older people by raising awareness, education, promoting research and the collection and dissemination of information. Action on Elder Abuse operates a confidential helpline service, providing information and advice, as well as emotional support, if required.

Age Exchange Theatre Trust and Reminiscence Centre
11 Blackheath Village
London SE3 9LA
Tel: 020 8318 9105
Fax: 020 8318 0060
Email: age-exchange@lewisham.gov.uk
Age Exchange is based at the Reminiscence Centre, a hands-on museum of objects from the 1930s and 1940s, which is open to the public. It runs reminiscence training days and is also involved in other aspects of reminiscence work, including theatre, publishing, exhibitions, workshops and intergenerational projects.

Alzheimer's Society
10 Greencoat Place
London SW1P 1PH
Tel: 020 7306 0606
Fax: 020 7306 0808
Helpline: 0845 300 0336 (local call rates)
Freephone information: 0800 027 2627
Email: Info@alzheimers.org.uk

Information, support and advice about caring for someone with Alzheimer's disease. Publishes a wide range of information sheets and other publication. Can also direct you to regional and local groups in England, Wales and Northern Ireland.

Alzheimer Scotland – Action on Dementia
22 Drumsheugh Gardens
Edinburgh EH3 7RN
Tel: 0131 243 1453
Fax: 0131 243 1450
Dementia helpline: 0808 808 3000
Email: alzheimer@alzscot.org

Information and support for people with dementia and their carers in Scotland. Supports a network of carers' support groups.

Dementia Services Development Centre (DSDC)
University of Stirling
Stirling FK9 4LA
Tel: 01786 467740
Fax: 01786 466846
Email: m.t.marshall@stir.ac.uk
Website: www.stir.ac.uk/dsdc

The Dementia Services Development Centre Network is a forum for existing and developing DSDCs in the UK. Based on the successful model pioneered at Stirling University, each Centre exists to provide services and information in a specified geographical area on all aspects of dementia, and dementia service provision to commissioners, service providers and policy makers. Operational Centres are located in:

Newcastle 0191 256 3318; Manchester 0161 275 5682; Oxford 01865 383706; Bristol 0117 975 4863; Wolverhampton 01902 575056; Wales 01248 383719 (Bangor) or 029 2049 4952 (Cardiff); London 020 8348 5231.

A centre also exists for Ireland, based in Dublin. If calling from the UK, dial 003531 453 7941 ext 2035.

Bradford Dementia Group
School of Health Studies
University of Bradford
West Yorkshire BD5 0BB
Tel: 01274 233996/236454
Fax: 01274 236395

Public Guardianship Office (formerly the Public Trust Office)
Stewart House
24 Kingsway
London WC2B 6JX
Tel: 020 7664 7300
Fax: 020 7664 7702

(It was formally announced in January 2001 that the Public Guardianship Office will be located at Archway Tower, Archway, North London. The anticipated time for relocation is late 2001/early 2002.)

For information about taking over the affairs of someone who is mentally incapacitated in England or Wales. In Scotland, enquiries should be addressed to the Public Guardian, Hadrian House, Callander Business Park, Falkirk FK1 1XR. Tel: 01324 678300. Website: scotcourts.gov.uk/. In Northern Ireland, enquiries should be addressed to The Office of Care and Protection, Royal Courts of Justice, PO Box 410, Chichester Street, Belfast BT1 3JF.

Speechmark Publishing Ltd
Telford Road
Bicester
Oxon OX26 4LQ
Tel: 01869 244644
Fax: 01869 320040
Email: info@speechmark.net

Produces a range of resources, under the Winslow brand, suitable for use with people with dementia.

About Age Concern

Dementia Care is one of a wide range of publications produced by Age Concern England, the National Council on Ageing. Age Concern works on behalf of all older people and believes later life should be fulfilling and enjoyable. For too many this is impossible. As the leading charitable movement in the UK concerned with ageing and older people, Age Concern finds effective ways to change that situation.

Where possible, we enable older people to solve problems themselves, providing as much or as little support as they need. A network of local Age Concerns, supported by 250,000 volunteers, provides community-based services such as lunch clubs, day centres and home visiting.

Nationally, we take a lead role in campaigning, parliamentary work, policy analysis, research, specialist information and advice provision, and publishing. Innovative programmes promote healthier lifestyles and provide older people with opportunities to give the experience of a lifetime back to their communities.

Age Concern is dependent on donations, covenants and legacies.

Age Concern England
1268 London Road
London SW16 4ER
Tel: 020 8765 7200
Fax: 020 8765 7211

Age Concern Scotland
113 Rose Street
Edinburgh EH2 3DT
Tel: 0131 220 3345
Fax: 0131 220 2779

Age Concern Cymru
4th Floor
1 Cathedral Road
Cardiff CF1 9SD
Tel: 029 2037 1566
Fax: 029 2039 9562

Age Concern Northern Ireland
3 Lower Crescent
Belfast BT7 1NR
Tel: 028 9024 5729
Fax: 028 9023 5497

Publications from Age Concern Books

Reminiscence and Recall: (2nd edition)
A guide to good practice
Faith Gibson

Completely revised and updated, this edition includes new guidance on working with people with dementia, international developments and creative communications. Packed with detailed advice on planning and running successful reminiscence work, other topics include:

- why reminiscence work can be valuable;
- suggestions for themed topics;
- using visual, audio and tactile triggers;
- planning and running a reminiscence group;
- intergenerational and life history work;
- working with people from different cultures.

This new edition provides advice and support to develop and maintain the very highest standards in reminiscence work.

£11.99 0-86242-253-1

Nutritional Care for Older People: A guide to good practice
June Copeman

Packed full of practical information and guidance, this book is designed to be used by all care staff concerned with food and nutrition and older people. Drawing on the latest scientific knowledge, national guidelines and accepted practice, this book will help staff develop and maintain the very best standards in all aspects of food management. Topics covered include:

- food environment and presentation;
- A-Z checklist of risk factors;
- frequency of meals and fluid intake;
- stimulating a small appetite;

- food and mental health issues;
- cultural and religious issues;
- menu planning and recipes;
- nutritional needs of people with specific illnesses.

Written by an experienced nutritionist, this book stresses throughout the importance of good nutrition to health. Staff involved in food planning and management in care homes, day centres and other community settings will find this book a vital source of guidance and support.

£14.99 0-86242-284-1

Culture, Religion and Patient Care in a Multi-ethnic Society
A handbook for professionals
Alix Henley and Judith Schott

This multi-disciplinary handbook aims to guide health professionals towards identifying and meeting the needs of different religious and cultural groups. It promotes the need for a framework of knowledge and ideas, as well as increased self-awareness. It will enable everyone involved in patient care to:

- explore aspects of patient care that may be affected by culture and religion;
- develop skills and awareness needed to communicate across cultural and language barriers;
- examine their own personal attitudes, assumptions and views about different cultural and religious groups;
- challenge institutional attitudes and working practices;
- fully understand the concepts of culture and 'race' and inequalities in health and healthcare provision;
- have a better understanding of the influence of culture and religion on everyday life, major events, and people's needs and reactions.

Rooted in the views and experiences of people of minority and cultural groups, this book provides professional carers with a unique blend of information, skills and awareness to enable them to understand and respond positively to the individual needs and wishes of patients.

£19.99 0-86242-231-0

Age Concern Training Packs

Age Concern Training Packs are ideal teaching tools for all care staff involved in the training and support of other staff. They enable trainers to effectively guide and reinforce skills and development by providing all the material necessary to run successful group training sessions.

The training packs:

- can be used either as an integrated or topic-led course;
- can be used again and again;
- can be used by inexperienced trainers;
- save time and money.

Most contain key point overhead transparencies, aims and objectives, teaching plans, group activities and support material and photocopiable handouts.

Packs already published:

The Everyday Affairs Training Pack: For use with care workers on basic legal and financial issues affecting older people
Toni Battison
£35.00 0-86242-291-4

The Reminiscence Trainer's Pack: For use in health, housing, social care and arts organisations; colleges, libraries and museums; volunteers' and carers' agencies
Faith Gibson
£35.00 0-86242-305-8

Accident Prevention in Residential and Nursing Homes: A training pack
Royal Society for the Prevention of Accidents (RoSPA)
£45.00 0-86242-290-6

The Successful Activity Co-ordinator Training Pack
Rosemary Hurtley and Jennifer Wenborn
£25.00 0-86242-265-5

Trained Nurse's Teaching Packs: For use in the workplace to educate nursing auxiliaries, health care assistants and social services care staff
Gill Early and Sarah Miller
Volume 1 £27.99   0-86242-213-2
Volume 2 £35.00   0-86242-286-8

Understanding Bereavement Training Pack: A guide for carers working with older people
Toni Battison
£35.00 0-86242-304-X

If you would like to order any of these titles, please write to the address below, enclosing a cheque or money order for the appropriate amount (plus £1.95 p&p) made payable to Age Concern England. Credit card orders may be made on 0870 44 22 044 (individuals); 0870 44 22 120 (AC federation, other organisations and institutions).

Age Concern Books
PO Box 232
Newton Abbot
Devon TQ12 4XQ

Age Concern Information Line/Factsheets subscription

Age Concern produces 44 comprehensive factsheets designed to answer many of the questions older people (or those advising them) may have. These include money and benefits, health, community care, leisure and education, and housing. For up to five free factsheets, telephone: 0800 00 99 66 (7am-7pm, seven days a week, every day of the year). Alternatively you may prefer to write to Age Concern, FREEPOST (SWB 30375), ASHBURTON, Devon TQ13 7ZZ.

For professionals working with older people, the factsheets are available on an annual subscription service, which includes updates throughout the year. For further details and costs of the subscription, please write to Age Concern at the above Freepost address.

Index